Current Cardiovascular Therapy

Series Editor
Juan Carlos Kaski

More information about this series at http://www.springer.com/
series/10472

Pasquale Perrone Filardi

Editor

ACEi and ARBS in Hypertension and Heart Failure

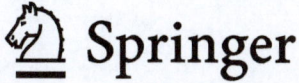 Springer

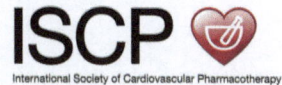
International Society of Cardiovascular Pharmacotherapy

Editor
Pasquale Perrone Filardi
Cardiology School
Federico II University of Naples
Naples, Italy

ISBN 978-3-319-09787-9   ISBN 978-3-319-09788-6 (eBook)
DOI 10.1007/978-3-319-09788-6
Springer Cham Heidelberg New York Dordrecht London

Library of Congress Control Number: 2014951210

Printed on acid-free paper

Springer is part of Springer Science+Business Media (www.springer.com)

Preface

The renin-angiotensin-aldosterone system has long been recognized to play a pivotal role in the pathogenesis of ischemic cardiovascular diseases and heart failure, and drugs that antagonize angiotensin II effects, namely ACE-inhibitors and AT1 receptor antagonists, are key in the therapy of patients affected by these conditions. These drugs have also demonstrated to reduce cardiovascular events in patients at high risk but without previous history of cardiovascular disease.

This book, along the aims of the International Society of Cardiovascular Pharmacotherapy, provides a comprehensive overview of the use of ACE-inhibitors and AT1 receptor antagonists in patients with common cardiovascular diseases, including hypertension and heart failure. Thus, the pharmacodynamic and pharmacokinetic properties of these classes of drugs are analyzed and discussed along with evidence coming from clinical studies that supports Guidelines recommendations. In particular, the book is covering clinical evidence on the benefit of these therapies in special patient populations, including patients with chronic kidney disease, diabetes mellitus and organ damage in whom renin-angiotensin system blockers are mandatorily recommended by Guidelines.

The purpose is to summarize, in a clear and updated fashion authored by world experts in the field, evidence based information on two among the most widespread cardiovascular classes of drugs to help physicians and healthcare professionals, particularly young doctors and trainees, deliver the most appropriate therapy to their patients.

Naples, Italy   Pasquale Perrone Filardi

Contents

Contents

Contributors

Editor
Pasquale Perrone Filardi Cardiology School, Federico II
University of Naples, Naples, Italy

Authors
Claudio Borghi Cattedra di Medicina Interna, Ospedale
S.Orsola.Malpighi, Bologna, Italy

Department of Medicine University of Bologna, Bologna, Italy

Eugenio Cosentino Department of Medicine, University of
Bologna, Bologna, Italy

Filippo Del Corso Department of Medicine, University of
Bologna, Bologna, Italy

Simone Faenza Department of Medicine, University of
Bologna, Bologna, Italy

Panagiotis I. Georgianos, M.D. Section of Nephrology and
Hypertension, 1st Department of Medicine, Aristotle University
of Thessaloniki, AHEPA University Hospital, Thessaloniki,
Greece

Athanasios J. Manolis, M.D., Ph.D. Department of
Cardiology, Asklepeion General Hospital, Athens, Greece

Carmine Morisco Dipartimento di Scienze Mediche
Traslazionali e Dipartimento di Scienze Biomediche Avanzate,
Università FEDERICO II Napoli, Naples, Italy

Giuseppe M.C. Rosano, M.D., Ph.D., FESC, FACC Department of Medical Sciences, Centre for Clinical and Basic Research, IRCCS San Raffaele Pisana, Rome, Italy

Cardiovascular and Cell Science Institute, St Georges University, London, UK

Pantelis A. Sarafidis, M.D., M.Sc., Ph.D. Department of Nephrology, "Hippokration" General Hospital, Aristotle University of Thessaloniki, Thessaloniki, Greece

Ilaria Spoletini, Ph.D. Department of Medical Sciences, Centre for Clinical and Basic Research, IRCCS San Raffaele Pisana, Rome, Italy

Bruno Trimarco Dipartimento di Scienze Mediche Traslazionali e Dipartimento di Scienze Biomediche Avanzate, Università FEDERICO II Napoli, Naples, Italy

Cristiana Vitale, M.D., Ph.D. Department of Medical Sciences, Centre for Clinical and Basic Research, IRCCS San Raffaele Pisana, Rome, Italy

Laboratory of Vascular Physiology, IRCCS San Raffaele, London, UK

Pantelis E. Zebekakis, M.D., Ph.D. Section of Nephrology and Hypertension, 1st Department of Medicine, Aristotle University of Thessaloniki, AHEPA University Hospital, Thessaloniki, Greece

Chapter 1
Angiotensin Converting Enzyme Inhibitors and AT1 Antagonists for Treatment of Hypertension

Carmine Morisco and Bruno Trimarco

Essential hypertension is the major cardiovascular risk factor. The main objective of treatment of essential hypertension is represented by long-term reduction of cardiovascular (CV) risk [59]. This goal can be achieved through the control of blood pressure (BP) values, the prevention of hypertension-related target organ damage (TOD) and metabolic complication, and reduction of CV events. During the last 25 years has emerged that the dysregulation of rennin-angiotensin-system (RAS) plays a pivotal role not only in the genesis of hypertension, but also in the development of TOD, diabetes, obesity, atherosclerosis and their complications. In fact, it has been documented that angiotensin II (Ang II), the effector of RAS, is involved in the regulation of endothelial function, tissue remodeling, inflammation, oxidative stress, differentiation of adipocytes, glucose metabolism and electrolytes homeostasis. Therefore, it does not surprise if the principal

C. Morisco • B. Trimarco (✉)
Dipartimento di Scienze Mediche Traslazionali e Dipartimento di Scienze Biomediche Avanzate, Università FEDERICO II Napoli, Naples, Italy
e-mail: trimarco@unina.it

© Springer International Publishing Switzerland 2015
P. Perrone Filardi (ed.), *ACEi and ARBS in Hypertension and Heart Failure*, Current Cardiovascular Therapy 5,
DOI 10.1007/978-3-319-09788-6_1

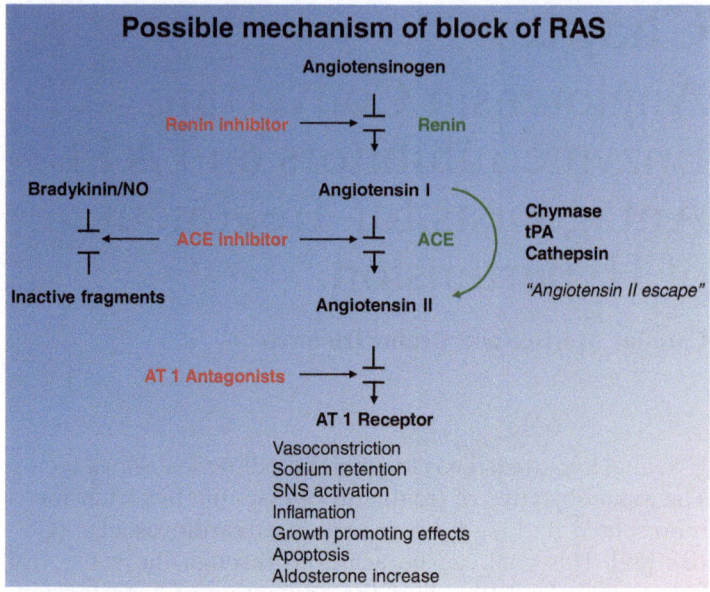

Fig. 1.1 Distinct pharmacological approach to bock the renin-angiotensin system (RAS)

interventional trials have demonstrated that the blocking of the RAS, obtained either with angiotensin converting enzyme (ACE)-inhibitors, or with the type 1 Ang II (AT_1) receptors blockers (ARBs) (Fig. 1.1), reduce the incidence of CV events in hypertensive and high CV risk patients. ACE-inhibitors block the conversion of angiotensin-I into Ang II reducing the circulating and local levels of Ang II. ACE-inhibitors also reduce the release of aldosterone and vaso-pressin, decrease the activity of sympathetic nervous system, as well as the trophic effects of Ang II on cardiac muscle and vessels. The inhibition of ACE produces also an increase in plasma bradykinin levels, which in turn, stimulates the type 2 bradykinin (B2) receptors leading to the release of nitric oxide (NO), and vasoactive prostaglandins (prostacyclin and prostaglandin E2). These biological effects are translated in several pharmacological actions consisting in the reduction of BP, in the decrease of plasma levels of epinephrine, norepinephrine and vasopressin, in the interference with development of vascular and cardiac hypertrophy and extracellular matrix proliferation, in the decrease renal vascular resistances and increase renal blood flow, which in turn, promotes Na^+ and water excretion, in the modulation of fibrinolytic balance resulting in antithrombotic effect.

AT_1 receptors belong to the superfamily of G-protein–coupled receptors that contain seven trans-membrane regions and are localized in the kidney, heart, vascular smooth muscle cells, brain, adrenal gland, platelets, adipocytes, and placenta. The AT_1 receptor mediates most of the detrimental effects of Ang II on cardiovascular system. In particular, their stimulation induces vasoconstriction, increases Na^+ retention, and endothelin secretion, enhances vasopressin release, activates sympathetic nervous activity, promotes cardiomyocytes hypertrophy, stimulates vascular and cardiac fibrosis, increases myocardial contractility, induces arrhythmias, stimulates plasminogen activator inhibitor 1, and stimulates superanoxide formation. ARBs act by blocking the AT_1 receptors and thus, prevent the pathophysiological effects mediated by the binding of Ang II to the AT_1 receptor. Moreover, as a consequence of AT_1 blockade, ARBs increase Ang II levels above baseline. Increased plasma levels of Ang II result in unopposed stimulation of the AT_2 receptors. It has been proposed that stimulation of AT_2 receptors exerts an important role in counterbalancing some of the detrimental effects of Ang II mediated by AT_1 receptors, such as inhibition of cell growth, promotion of cell differentiation, and synthesis of NO. Finally, for some ARBs has been documented an agonist action on PPAR-γ receptors. These biological effects are translated in different pharmacological actions such as prevention of hypertension-induced TOD, of hypertension-associated diseases such as diabetes, atherosclerosis, and renal disease; interestingly, these effects appear to be potentially independent from ARBs-induced BP reduction.

RAS Inhibition and Blood Pressure Lowering

The relation between BP and CV events is a continuous phenomenon without threshold [52] The RAS plays a pivotal role in the regulation of BP; therefore, drugs affecting RAS like ACE and ARBs are largely used for BP control and for management of CV risk. The CAPPP study was the first prospective, randomised intervention trial aimed to evaluate the effects of ACE inhibition and conventional therapy on cardiovascular morbidity and mortality in patients with essential hypertension. This study enrolled 10,985 patients: 5,492 patients assigned captopril and 5,493 assigned conventional therapy; the two treatment regimens had the same effect on blood pressure, and incidence of major cardiovascular events [30]. The interpretation of the results of this study was that an antihypertensive regimen based on ACE inhibitors was as effective as conventional treatment with diuretics, β-blockers, or both in prevention of cardiovascular morbidity and mortality. Similarly the STOP-2 study [29] showed in elderly patients that the incidence of cardiovascular events was similar in elderly hypertensives randomized to a calcium antagonist, an ACE inhibitor, or conventional treatment with a diuretic or a β-blocker, and decrease in blood pressure was of major importance for the prevention of cardiovascular events. ARBs represent a class of effective and well tolerated orally active antihypertensive drugs. The antihypertensive effects of the ARBs have been demonstrated by many interventional studies. In a meta-analysis Conlin et al. analyzed 43 randomized, controlled clinical trials comparing the antihypertensive effects of ARBs (losartan, valsartan, irbesartan, and candesartan) with placebo, other antihypertensive classes, and each other. The analysis included 11,281 patients treated with ARBs showed that the weighted average of diastolic and systolic blood pressure (BP) reductions and responder rates among agents were comparable, irrespective of starting doses, monotherapy dose titration, and combination therapy with hydrochlorothiazide (HCTZ) [15]. Available data indicate that both ACE-inhibitors and ARBs are comparable to other antihypertensive agents in lowering blood pressure: However, these two classes of drugs are more effective, compared to others antihypertensive drugs, in the prevention of metabolic abnormalities and sub-clinical organ damage.

RAS Inhibition and Hypertension-Related Metabolic Abnormalities

Essential hypertension often is associated with metabolic abnormalities which can exert a detrimental effects on the prognosis. Therefore, the prevention of diabetes, metabolic syndrome and dyslipidemias represents a key point of antihypertensive treatment. Inhibition of RAS has been demonstrate to have a favorable effect in the prevention of such abnormalities.

Dyslipidemias

Clinical evidence: Interventional studies have demonstrated that pharmacological interference of RAS, slightly improves the lipid profile in hypertensive patients. This beneficial action has been demonstrated for the different ARBs. In particular, Kyvelou et al. demonstrated, in a cohort of 2,438 hypertensive patients, followed for 6 months, that treatment with ARBs-based monotherapy induce a significant reduction of total and LDL-cholesterol, in addition increase HDL-cholesterol [50]. Furthermore, a sub-study of LIFE showed in hypertensive patients that, in comparison with atenolol-based, losartan-based regimen, induces a less decrease in HDL-C; and this pharmacological effect is associated with a better prognosis [66]. The authors speculated that less decrease in HDL-C may explain around one-third of the beneficial effect of losartan-based compared with atenolol-based antihypertensive treatment on composite end-point found in the LIFE study. The favorable effects on lipid profile have been documented for ARBs also when these are combined with antihypertensive drugs that aggravated metabolic profile. In particular, the Alpine Study showed that treatment with diuretics, if needed, in combination with a β-blocker was associated with a worsening of metabolic profile; this effect was not detected for patients treated with an ARB [55]. Some ARBs such as telmisartan and eprosartan, have been reported to stimulate peroxisome proliferator-activated receptor-γ (PPARγ) [82] and could thus improve insulin sensitivity [67]. This, indirectly could influence systemic lipid concentrations, so it is unclear whether the differences in results from clinical trials arise from these ancillary properties of RAS blockade. However, two studies failed to demonstrate the beneficial effects of ARBs on lipid profile in hypertensive patients. In particular Grassi et al. in the CROSS study evaluated in obese hypertensive individuals the antihypertensive, neuroadrenergic, and metabolic effects of an ARB in comparison with a diuretic. The results of this study showed that after 3 months of treatment, despite Candesartan improved insulin sensitivity had no effect on plasma levels of triglycerides, of HDL-cholesterol and of LDL-cholesterol [27]. More recently, Nishida et al. confirmed the observation of Grassi, demonstrating that in patients with mild to moderate hypertension Candesartan has no effect on plasma levels of triglycerides, of total and of LDL-cholesterol [65].

Experimental evidence: ANG II exerts several effects that influence atherogenic properties of cholesterol. In particular, it has been demonstrated that AT1A receptor deficiency had a striking effect in reducing hypercholesterolemia-induced atherosclerosis in LDL receptor-negative mice [19]. Moreover, in this model hypercholesterolemia was associated with increased systemic angiotensinogen and angiotensin peptides, which were reduced in AT1A receptor-deficient mice, suggesting that LDL cholesterol contributes to development of atherosclerosis through a RAS-dependent mechanism. Moreover, it has been reported in primary cultures of human monocyte-macrophages, that the pro-atherogenic effects of ANG II are related to the property of ANG II to upregulate the expression of Acyl-CoA: cholesterol acyltransferase-1

(ACAT1) [41]. This enzyme converts free cholesterol into esters for storage in lipid droplets. This process could promote foam cell formation, and increase cholesterol content of atherosclerotic lesions. Finally, Several studies have reported that ANG II increased the oxidation of LDL in macrophage cell lines as well as mouse peritoneal macrophages, possibly through activation of NADPH oxidase [42]. Altogether these observations are consistent with the notion that ANG II may influence the atherogenic properties of cholesterol without necessarily changing the blood concentrations [69]. Interestingly, cholesterol is capable to regulate RAS. In particular, it has been demonstrated the capability of LDL cholesterol to increase AT_1 receptor gene expression on vascular smooth muscle cells [64] as well as, oxidized LDL can also increase AT1 receptor gene expression in human coronary artery endothelial cells [54]. Together, these results clearly demonstrate a cross-talk between hypercholesterolemia and RAS in the development of atherosclerosis.

Metabolic Syndrome and Obesity

Clinical evidence: Metabolic syndrome (MetS) has been defined in different ways, and it is a risk factor for development of atherosclerosis and occurrence of CV events. A feature of MetS is the constellation of risk factors including abdominal adiposity, impaired fasting glucose, hypertension, and dyslipidemia. Moreover, obesity also predisposes to CV disease and often is associated with other abnormalities of the MetS. In particular, adipose tissue acts as an endocrine organ, secreting hormones and other substances that create a proinflammatory state and promote formation of atherosclerotic plaques [51]. In the last years many interventional studies specifically addressed the effects of RAS inhibition/antagonism in metabolic syndrome. In particular the hemodynamic and metabolic effects of two ARBs were particularly evaluated: telmisartan and irbesartan. These molecules activates effect on the activity of peroxisome proliferator-activated receptor gamma, a well-known target for insulin-sensitizing antidiabetic drugs. In particular, the ISLAND [87] study demonstrated that Administration of irbesartan and/or lipoic acid to patients with the metabolic syndrome improves endothelial function and reduces proinflammatory markers, factors that are implicated in the pathogenesis of atherosclerosis The OLAS study evaluated the effects of different treatments with olmesartan/amlodipine and olmesartan/hydrochlorothiazide on inflammatory and metabolic parameters in nondiabetic hypertensive patients with MetS [60]. This study showed that olmesartan-based combinations were effective, but the amlodipine combination resulted in metabolic and anti-inflammatory effects that may have advantages over the hydrochlorothiazide combination. More recently, it was demonstrated the capability of telmisartan to activates PPARγ in circulating monocytes of patients with the metabolic syndrome [6]. Many intervention trials have not been designed specifically for obese hypertensive patients, and only few studies have specifically addressed the use of ACE-inhibitors or ARBs in these patients. For instance, the TROPHY study, was a multicenter, double-blind trial that evaluated the efficacy and safety of the lisinopril, against the hydrochlorothiazide, in obese, hypertensive patients [71]. The results of this study showed that, despite similar reductions in office systolic BP and diastolic BP with lisinopril or hydrochlorothiazide, treatment with angiotensin-converting enzyme inhibitors has a greater efficacy as monotherapy at lower doses compared with thiazide diuretics.

Experimental evidence: Several mechanisms account for the association between MetS and increased risk of atherosclerotic CV events. For instance, there is growing evidence that RAS, through Ang II, is involved not only in the pathogenesis of hypertension and atherosclerosis, but also plays a role in the development of insulin resistance. Moreover, it has also demonstrated that activation of the RAS in adipose tissue represents an important mechanism that account for the link between obesity and hypertension [20]. Adipose tissue is an important production site of angiotensinogen, and it has been reported a correlation between plasma level of angiotensinogen, blood pressure, and body mass index [74]. Moreover, in obese Zucker rats it has been documented an increase higher than 50 % of gene expression of angiotensinogen, in adipose tissue compared with lean rats [39]. Interestingly, it has been also demonstrated that Ang II is implicated in the regulation of lipid synthesis and storage in the adipocytes [20], as well as, in adipocyte growth and differentiation [2]. In addition, it has been documented that the AT_1 receptor, and ACE genes were found to be upregulated in the adipose tissue of hypertensive patients with obesity [25]. Altogether these experimental evidence suggest a strong relationship between RAS and regulation of functional activity of adipose tissue, this phenomenon could be involved in the increase of both BP and CV risk.

Insulin Resistance and Diabetes

Clinical evidence: The beneficial effects of ACE inhibitors to improve insulin resistance are also evident from several observational and interventional studies in human subjects with hypertension and type 2 diabetes. For instance, in the Captopril Prevention Project (CAPPP) [30] and the Heart Outcomes Prevention Evaluation (HOPE) study [105], two large prospective studies involving hypertensive subjects at risk for developing type 2 diabetes, there was a lesser incidence of newly-diagnosed type 2 diabetes in those subjects who received an ACE inhibitor (either captopril or ramipril) compared to the respective placebo control groups. More consistently, in 2005, it has been published a meta-analysis of 12 randomized controlled clinical trials of ACE inhibitors or ARBs to evaluate the efficacy of these medications in diabetes prevention. This meta-analysis, involving 72,333 nondiabetic patients (approximately 338,000 patient-years of follow-up), with mean duration of follow-up ranged from 1 to 6.1 years, showed that ACE inhibitors or ARBs produced a highly significant 25 % reduction (or a decrease from 17.4 to

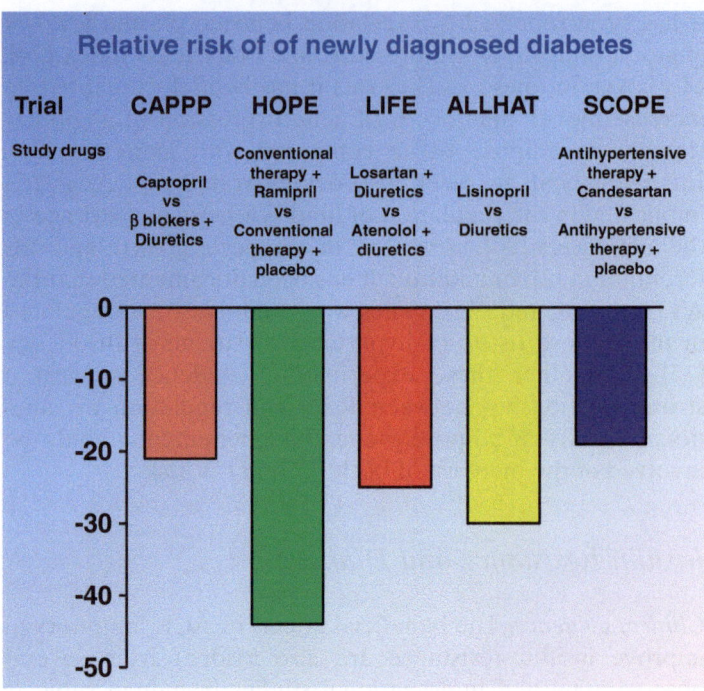

FIG. 1.2 Results of principal intervention trial with renin-angiotensin system (RAS) inhibitors on new diagnosis of diabetes

14.3 cases per 1,000 patient-years) in the incidence of new-onset diabetes [1]. The clinical implications of this meta-analysis are important because the development of diabetes is associated with insulin resistance. Therefore, it is possible to speculate that the inhibition of RAS by both ACE inhibitors or by AT 1 receptor antagonists ameliorates insulin sensitivity (Fig. 1.2). The mechanisms of action whereby these classes of drugs improve insulin sensitivity are complex and multifactorial. In particular, ACE inhibitors not only block the conversion of angiotensin I to angiotensin II, but also increase bradykinin levels through inhibition of kininase II-mediated degradation. The higher kinin levels lead to an increased production of prostaglandins (prostaglandin E1 and prostaglandin E2) and nitric oxide, which improve exercise-induced glucose metabolism and muscle sensitivity to insulin [24], resulting in enhanced insulin-mediated glucose uptake. Furthermore, the peripheral vasodilatory actions of ACE inhibitors and ARBs lead to an improvement in skeletal muscle blood flow, the primary target for insulin action and an important determinant of glucose uptake. This effectively increases the surface area for glucose exchange between the vascular bed and skeletal muscles. Clinical evidence supporting this effect has been provided by Morel et al. [61], who have demonstrated improved insulin sensitivity when enalapril was given for 12 weeks to 14 obese, hypertensive, and dyslipidemic patients. A similar effect has also been reported with captopril [68]. However, it should be underlined that this action can not be considered the main mechanism that account for the increase of insulin sensitivity because this effect is not shared by drugs that acts as vasodilators like hydralazine. Moreover, the protection against the development of insulin resistance may be partially due to a regulation of adipocyte function. It has been demonstrated that increased levels of Ang II inhibit pre-adipocyte differentiation into mature adipocytes, and this impairs the fat cells' ability to store fat. This, in turn results in shunting of fats to the liver, skeletal muscle, and pancreas, which worsens insulin resistance. Reducing Ang II levels with an ACE inhibitor or blocking the angiotensin II receptor type 1 with an ARB may promote differentiation of pre-adipocytes to mature adipocytes, which serve as a sump for fat. In addition, redistribution of the lipids from the peripheral tissues would improve insulin sensitivity [84]. Another mechanism that accounts for the favorable effect of ARBs and ACE inhibitors on insulin sensitivity relates to a possible protective effect on the pancreatic beta cell, through inhibiting the vasoconstrictive effect of angiotensin II in the pancreas and increasing islet blood flow [10], which could improve insulin release by beta cells. Telmisartan, an ARB, has been shown to act as a peroxisome proliferator-activated receptor

(PPAR)-gamma agonist, similar to the thiazolidinediones rosiglitazone and pioglitazone, which preserve pancreatic beta-cell function [82]. Peroxisome proliferator–activated receptor γ is a transcription factor that controls the gene expression of several key enzymes of glucose metabolism and thereby increases insulin sensitivity.

Experimental and clinical studies suggest that blocking the effects of Ang II (through ACE inhibition or ARBs) increases insulin sensitivity, skeletal muscle glucose transport, and pancreatic blood flow, which may contribute to the prevention of diabetes mellitus. Therefore, ACE inhibitors or ARBs represent the logical first-line anti-hypertensive agent in patients with impaired fasting glucose or metabolic syndrome for multiple reasons, including the reduction in risk of progression to overt type 2 diabetes. Even in patients without diabetes or metabolic syndrome, what was previously thought to be a "high-normal" blood pressure ($\geq$130/80 to 139/89 mmHg) is associated with an increased risk of adverse cardiovascular events [100].

Experimental evidence: In vivo and in vitro studies have shown that Ang II stimulation also induces insulin resistance. Overactivity of the RAS observed in cardiovascular diseases is likely to impair insulin signaling and contribute to insulin resistance. Actually, Ang II acting through the AT1 receptor inhibits the actions of insulin in vascular tissue, in part, by interfering with insulin signaling through PI3K and downstream Akt signaling pathways via generation of reactive oxygen species (ROS) by NADPH oxidase. ROS are important intracellular second messengers that activate many downstream signaling molecules, such as phosphotyrosine phosphatases (PTPase) and protein tyrosine kinases. PTPases are critical regulators of tyrosine phosphorylation-dependent signaling, and tyrosine dephosphorylation by PTPases may play a crucial role in Ang II-induced insulin resistance. Several PTPs have been implicated in the Ang II-induced dephosphorylation of insulin receptor. However, the most convincing data, support a critical role for PTP-1B in insulin action. Actually, PTP-1B knockout mice display increased insulin sensitivity and maintain euglycemia (in the fed state) with one-half the level of insulin observed in wild-type littermates. Interestingly, these mice are also resistant to diet-induced obesity when fed a high-fat diet.

Recent studies have demonstrated that the generation of ROS is implicated in the Ang II-induced insulin resistance. In this regard it has been demonstrated that in vascular smooth muscle cells isolated from rat thoracic aorta Ang II profoundly decreases IRS-1 protein levels via ROS-mediated phosphorylation of IRS-1 on Ser307 and subsequent proteasome-dependent degradation. The key role of ROS in the pathogenesis of Ang II-induced insulin resistance has been also confirmed by in vivo studies. In particular, in rats chronic infusion of Ang II reduced insulin-induced glucose uptake during hyperinsulinemic-euglycemic clamp, and increased plasma cholesterylester hydroperoxide levels, indicating an increased oxidative stress. Treatment with tempol, a superoxide dismutase mimetic, normalized plasma cholesterylester hydroperoxide levels in AII-infused rats. In addition, tempol normalized insulin resistance in AII-infused rats, as well as enhanced insulin-induced PI 3-kinase activation, suggesting that Ang II-induced insulin resistance can be restored by removing the oxidative stress. On the other hand, in the endothelial cells, Ang II induces insulin resistance through the phosphorylation of IRS-1 at Ser312 and Ser616 via JNK- and ERK1/2-dependent mechanisms, respectively. This impairs the interaction of IRS-1 with the p85 regulatory subunit of PI 3-kinase and compromises the insulin vasodilatory signaling pathway involving PI 3-kinase/Akt/eNOS. Altogether, these observations provide clear insight into the mechanisms of Ang II–induced insulin resistance. ACE inhibitors decrease the conversion of angiotensin I to Ang II, in addition, via the inhibition of the kininase II breakdown, enhance the circulating level of the bradykinin (Fig. 1.3). There are several experimental data indicating that these changes in Ang II and bradykinin improve skeletal muscle glucose metabolism. In particular, there are experimental studies performed in animal models of hypertension and

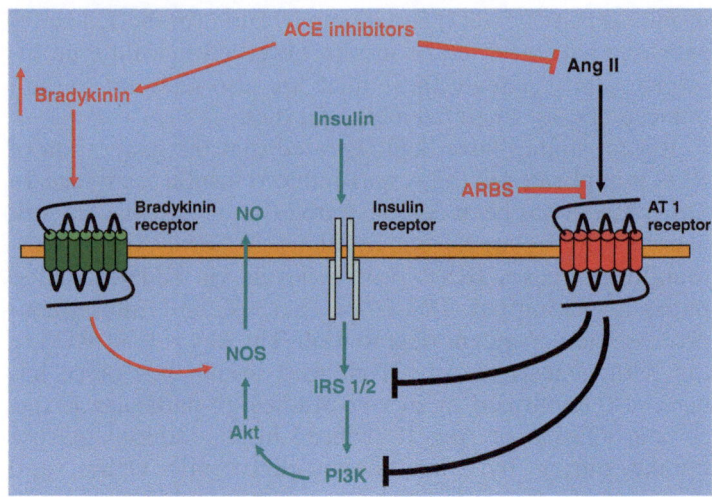

Fig. 1.3 Molecular mechanisms that account for improvement of insulin sensitivity following renin-angiotensin system inhibition

insulin resistance which have demonstrated that acute and chronic administration of ACE inhibitors can improve insulin action on whole-body and skeletal muscle glucose disposal. In particular, it has been demonstrated in 20-month-old rats that the acute oral administration of the ACE inhibitor captopril enhances whole-body insulin action on glucose disappearance during an intravenous insulin tolerance test by modulating the early steps of insulin signaling, and that this effect may be simulated by the administration of bradykinin [11]. Moreover, the acute infusion of captopril to obese Zucker rats, a rodent model of insulin resistance, glucose intolerance, and dyslipidemia, enhances insulin sensitivity during a euglycemic, hyperinsulinemic clamp [4]. A similar response to an acute captopril infusion has been observed in an insulin resistant diabetic dog model using this euglycemic, hyperinsulinemic clamp technique [98]. In addition to acute administration, also chronic treatment with ACE inhibitors has been demonstrated to enhance glucose tolerance in animal models of insulin resistance. In fact, it has been shown that chronic administration of ACE inhibitors to obese Zucker rats elicits an increase in whole-body insulin action. Chronic oral treatment of obese Zucker rats with the ACE inhibitors captopril [18], or trandolapril [89] causes substantial improvements in whole-body insulin sensitivity, assessed during an oral glucose tolerance test, and these ACE inhibitor-mediated improvements in whole-body insulin sensitivity are associated with decreases in plasma insulin and amelioration of dyslipidemia. Chronic administration of an ACE inhibitor to a mouse model of type 2 diabetes (KK-Ay) also significantly improves whole-body glucose tolerance and insulin sensitivity [85].

Skeletal muscle is an important locus of ACE inhibitor action in rodent models of insulin resistance and hypertension. Acute in vivo administration of the ACE inhibitors captopril [31] or trandolapril [36] significantly enhances insulin-mediated glucose transport activity in skeletal muscle in the obese Zucker rat. Skeletal muscle is not the only muscle tissue in which ACE inhibitors can beneficially modulate glucose metabolism. Rett et al. [72] have demonstrated using the perfused Langendorff preparation that the acute administration of active ACE inhibitor metabolite phosphorylate can significantly increase insulin-stimulated glucose transport activity in cardiac muscle of the obese Zucker rat, and that this effect can be mimicked by administration of bradykinin.

RAS Inhibition and Hypertension-Related TOD

Subclinical organ damage is an important determinant of CV risk in essential hypertension, and represents a key target of antihypertensive therapy. Interestingly, Ang II plays a critical role in the pathogenesis of TOD (Fig. 1.4). Thus, RAS blockade should be considered as first choice therapy of hypertensive patients with evidence of TOD.

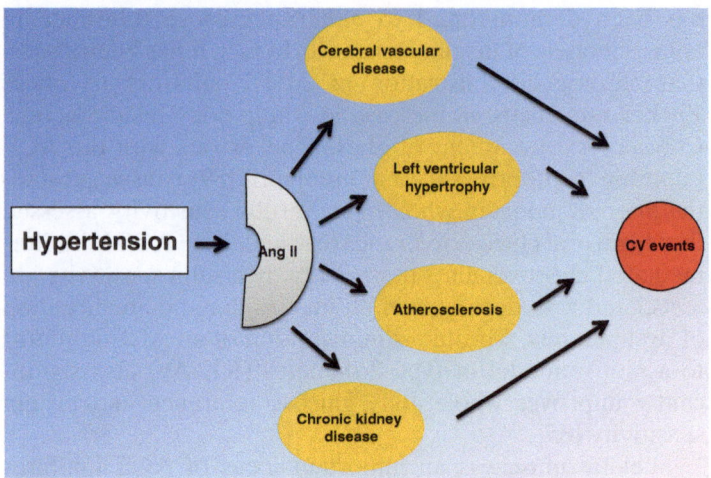

FIG. 1.4 Central role of angiotensin II (Ang II) in the pathogenesis of target organ damage and cardiovascular (CV) events in essential hypertension

Left Ventricular Hypertrophy

Clinical evidence: Left ventricular hypertrophy (LVH) is an independent risk factor for morbidity and mortality for CV diseases. BP is an important determinant of LVH, and a substantial percentage of patients with hypertension develop this complication. Several studies have analyzed the effects of different classes of antihypertensive drugs on LVH. The first meta-analysis aimed to assess the ability of various antihypertensive agents to reduce left ventricular hypertrophy was published in 1996 by Schmieder et al. [81]. This analysis considered 39 double-blind, randomized, controlled clinical studies with parallel-group design. After adjustment for different durations of treatment, left ventricular mass decreased by 13 % with ACE inhibitors, 9 % with calcium channel blockers, 6 % with beta-blockers, and 7 % with diuretics. There was a significant difference between drug classes (P < .01): ACE inhibitors reduced left ventricular mass more than beta-blockers (significant, P < .05) and diuretics

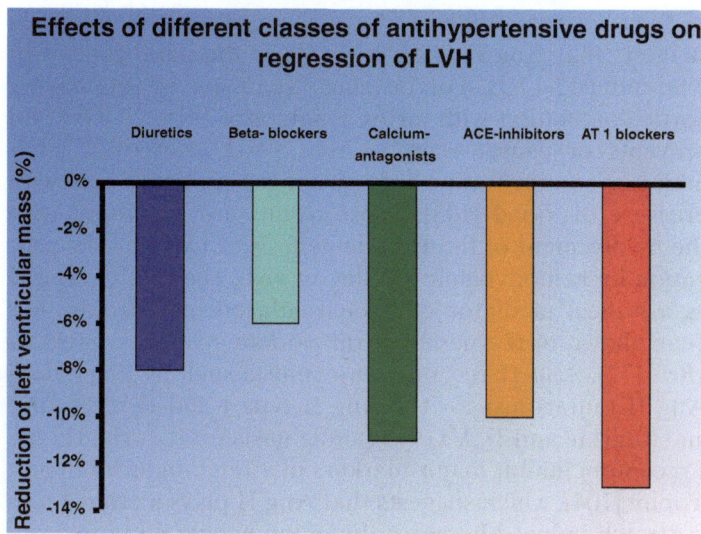

FIG. 1.5 Effects of different classes of antihypertensive drugs on regression of left ventricular hypertrophy (LVH)

(tendency, $P = .08$), suggesting the ACE inhibitors as first-line drugs to reduce LVH. In 2003 was published a further meta-analysis that added also ARBs-based clinical trials. This analysis considered a total 80 studies with more than 4,000 patients [44]. The principal finding of this analysis was that ARBs, calcium antagonists, and ACE-inhibitors were the most effective drug classes for reducing left ventricular mass in patients with essential hypertension (Fig. 1.5). In 2009 a metaregression-analysis assessed, in patients with essential hypertension, the predictor of the regression of LVH among the principal classes of antihypertensive drugs [21]. This analysis considered of 75 prospective, randomized comparative trials, including 6,001 patients, with a median study duration of 6 months. The main result of this analysis showed that ARBs induce larger regression of LVH. These studies indicate that RAS inhibition with both ACE-inhibitors or ARBs represents a valid pharmacologic strategy to prevent or reduce LVH.

Experimental evidence: Several experimental evidence suggests that Ang II has a key role in the pathogenesis of load-induced LVH. For instance, treatment of rats having aortic coarctation with an ACE inhibitor [9] or ARBs [46] prevents or causes regression of LVH. Moreover, ACE inhibitor administration also prolongs survival of rats with pressure overload [103]. These results are consistent with the involvement of the RAS in genesis of LVH and its activation by hemodynamic loading in vivo. The role of Ang II as a critical mediator of stretch-induced hypertrophy has been shown in the neonatal rat cardiac myocyte system *in vitro* [77]. Ang II receptor antagonists such as [Sar1 Ile8] Ang II (antagonist for the Ang II type I and II receptors) and losartan and TCV11974 (antagonists for the Ang II type I receptor) inhibit major markers of stretch-induced hypertrophy [104], which suggests that Ang II plays a critical role in stretch-induced hypertrophy in the neonatal rat myocyte culture system [79]. Several lines of *in vivo* evidence suggest that the cardiac RAS is upregulated chronically in load-induced hypertrophy. mRNA expression of angiotensinogen, renin, ACE, and Ang II receptor are all upregulated in cardiac hypertrophy caused by pressure overload and ischemia [93]. The upregulation of the cardiac RAS was also observed in mechanical stretch of neonatal rat cardiac myocytes *in vitro* [79]. Treatment of cultured cardiac myocytes with exogenous Ang II also upregulates mRNA expression of angiotensinogen, renin, and ACE, but not Ang II receptor [86]. This suggests that mechanical stretch initially causes acute secretion of preformed Ang II and that secreted Ang II may initiate a positive feedback mechanism, thereby upregulating the local renin-angiotensin system over time. It is likely, however, that upregulation of the Ang II receptor by mechanical stretch is mediated by an Ang II-independent mechanism [78]. Further studies have demonstrated the molecular mechanism that account for Ang II-mediated development of LVH. In particular, Bendall et al. demonstrated, in transgenic mice lacking the gp91[phox] subunit of NADPH oxidase, that 2 week-stimulation of subpressor doses of Ang II stimulation failed to induce LVH, this was associated with inhibition to superoxide production [7]. The result of this study indicated that oxidative stress is centrally involved in the direct cardiac hypertrophic response to Ang II.

Chronic Kidney Disease

Clinical evidence: Development of chronic kidney disease (CKD) a common feature of essential hypertension. The renal damage, is characterized by a progressive loss of renal function, and, at the same time, increases cardiovascular risk. Ang II plays a key role in the pathogenesis of CKD in essential hypertension. In particular, excess of Ang II stimulation induces endothelial dysfunction, which, in the kidneys, can evolve in glomerulosclerosis, tubulointerstitial fibrosis and vascular sclerosis. In the absence of pharmacological intervention, these abnormalities are responsible of development of overt nephropathy that culminates in endstage of renal disease (ESRD). Clinical manifestations of hypertension-induced nephropathy are: presence of macroalbuminuria or proteinuria, decrease of glomerular filtration rate (GFR), increase in serum creatinine levels. Although achievement of a tight control of BP is important goal to prevent CKD, this strategy, alone, often is not enough to prevent the development and progression of CKD. The benefit of ACE inhibitor therapy in reducing proteinuria and the progression of CKD in non-diabetic patients are known since 1990s; similarly, beneficial effects has been demonstrated also for ARBs in nondiabetic nephropathies [95]. Thus, antihypertensive drugs that interfere with RAS confer additional renoprotective benefits compared with other classes of antihypertensive agents. The first convincing demonstration of the ability of ACE-inhibitors to interfere with the progression of CKD comes from the REIN study. This study showed that although BP control did not differ between the two treatment groups, patients who had proteinuria of ≥ 3 g/day and were treated with the ACE inhibitor showed a significant lower rate of decline in GFR and a reduced risk for doubling serum creatinine or end-stage renal failure as compared with patients who received conventional therapy [28]. The favorable effects of ACE-inhibitors [38] in the delay of CKD have been confirmed by several meta-analysis [37, 48]. The beneficial effects of many ARBs have been well documented in diabetic nephropathy. In fact, clinical trials with irbesartan, losartan, telmisartan and valsartan have been conducted in patients with type 2 diabetes and CKD. On the contrary, there are few clinical evidence of the nefroprotective effects of ARBs in patients with non-diabetic nephropathy. In details, The Japanese Losartan Therapy Intended for the Global Renal Protection in HyperTensive Patients (JLIGHT) study examined the effect of losartan in comparison with amlodipine after 12 months of treatment. This study showed that although losartan and amlodipine had a comparable antihypertensive effect, losaran based treatment significantly reduced the severity of proteinuria [34]. In addition, the Angiotensin II Receptor Antagonist Micardis in Isolated Systolic hypertension (ARAMIS) study compared the antihypertensive efficacy after 6 weeks of once-daily fixed doses of telmisartan 20, 40 or 80 mg versus hydrochlorothiazide 12.5 mg or placebo in patients (n = 1,039, aged 35–84 years) with isolated systolic hypertension. This study showed that, despite comparable reductions in systolic blood pressure with both drugs, telmisartan treatment significantly reduced urinary albumin excretion than hydrochlorothiazide [102].

Experimental evidence: In last years is has been demonstrated that CKD is characterized by of chronic inflammation associated with oxidative stress, endothelial dysfunction, and vascular calcification. Moreover, it has also been documented that Ang II regulates not only the hydro-saline homeostasis and peripheral vascular resistances but, exerts also a control on cell growth, inflammation, and fibrosis [75]. Together these experimental evidence indicate that Ang II plays a pivotal role in the genesis of CKD in essential hypertension by modulating the redox status and the immune system. In fact, Ang II increases tumor necrosis factor-production in the kidney, as well as, upregulates other proinflammatory mediators, including interleukin 6, monocyte chemotactic protein-1, and nuclear factor-B [94], resulting in a variety of glomerular insults. These results allow the hypothesize that Ang II is involved into the pathogenesis of CKD by modulating the activation and infiltration of immunocompetent cells There are several evidence showing that some of the beneficial effects of the RAS blockade may be related to anti-inflammatory properties of ACE-inhibitors and ARBs [91]. In particular, it has been reported in monocytes that exposure to captopril affects the cytokine-induced translocation of nuclear factor-kB translocation from the cytoplasm to the nucleus [3]. Furthermore, it has been reported in patients with ESRD, that ACE-inhibitor-based treatment reduces plasma levels of plasma levels of tumor necrosis factor-α and C-reactive protein [90].

Dual RAS Inhibition

Definitely, blockade of the RAS with obtained with either ACE-inhibitors or ARBs has been shown to reduce proteinuria and the decline of GFR. However, not all patients who are treated with ACEI or ARBs achieve a nefro-protective effect. This phenomenon might be explained by an incomplete blockade of RAS. In fact, different pathways (mainly chymases), especially during diabetic nephropathy, can account for Ang II synthesis. Therefore, treatment with combination of both ACEI and ARBs may have a synergistic effect on RAS blockade in prevention of kidney disease in hypertension. In the last decade, two studies that included a small number of patients reported in hypertensive patients the beneficial effects of dual RAS blockade. Then, the Cooperate study analyzed 263 patients with non-diabetic renal disease, randomly assigned to ARB (losartan, 100 mg daily), or ACE-inhibitor (trandolapril, 3 mg daily), or a combination of both drugs. The main result of this study was that combination treatment safely retarded the progression of non-diabetic renal disease compared with monotherapy [62]. In 2009 this study was retracted due to ethic concerns. The nefro-protective effects of dual bock of RAS were evaluated in two meta-analysis [12, 49] which showed of the favorable effects of combination therapy of ACE-inhibitor and ARBs to reduce proteinuria and to slow the progression of CKD. However, these actions were not confirmed by the ONTARGET study (ONTARGET [35]) in which patients were randomized to receive ACE-inhibitor (Ramipril 10 mg daily) or ARB (Telmisartan 80 mg daily) or both drugs. This study reported an increased incidence of dialysis, doubling of serum creatinine and of death during the combined therapy of ACE inhibitor and ARBs compared with a monotherapy alone; whereas albuminuria was best controlled by the dual RAS blockade. The main reason for this negative result could be identified in the very high risk of study population. Therefore, further trials that enroll patients with a lower cardiovascular risk are necessary to establish whether the combination of ACE inhibitor and ARBs is detrimental or beneficial on CKD.

Atherosclerosis

Clinical evidence: Essential hypertension is an established risk factor for the development of atherosclerosis. Both clinical and experimental evidence indicate that hypertension promotes and accelerates the atherosclerotic process through an Ang II mediated mechanisms; in particular, it has been demonstrated that Ang II inflammatory processes and oxidative stress that lead the formation of arterial lesions or plaques. Interference with RAS has been demonstrated to reduce the progression of the atherogenic process [23]. Although many patients included in the HOPE study were not affected by essential hypertension, this study demonstrated, in high risk patients, that addition of ramipril to the standard therapy significantly reduced the rate of the primary composite endpoint vs placebo (14.0 % vs 17.8 %; $P < 0.001$) [105]. Interestingly, in this study population, use of ramipril reduced not only the cardio- and cerebro-vascular events, but interfered also with the progression of atherosclerotic disease. In fact, SECURE study, substudy of the HOPE trial demonstrated that the rate of progression of the mean maximum carotid artery IMT was significantly lower in the ramipril 10 mg once-daily treatment group vs placebo ($P = 0.028$) over an average follow-up period of 4.5 years [57]. In hypertensive patients with and without diabetes it has been reported that candesartan [5] and losartan [88] respectively, slows the progression of carotid remodeling. Several studies have demonstrated the effect of RAS blockade on the mechanisms that are involved in the development and progression of atherosclerosis. In particular, it has been reported that candesartan significantly decreases plasma levels of plasminogen activator inhibitor type-1 (PAI-1), as well as monocyte chemoattractant protein-1 [45] and significantly reduces circulating levels of ICAM-1 and VCAM-1 [73]. Similar actions have been reported for irbesartan, valsartan and losartan. In addition, several studies have demonstrated that Olmesartan medoxomil-based therapies interferes with the vascular inflammation and progression of atherosclerosis not only in carotid, but also in coronary arteries. In particular, the OLIVUS showed that demonstrated that olmesartan medoxomil decreased the rate of coronary atheroma progression in patients with stable angina pectoris, independent of BP lowering [32].

Experimental evidence: Ang II plays a pivotal role not only in the development of atherosclerosis but also in the vulnerability of atherosclerotic plaques. In fact, It has been reported that Ang II regulates the gene expression and synthesis of adhesion molecule (VCAM-1, ICAM-1, P-selectin), cytokine, chemokine, and growth factor of the arterial wall. In addition, RAS positively regulates the complement system, resulting in vascular inflammation and mobilization/and activation of inflammatory cells. The RAS interferes also with coagulation cascade and platelet aggregation. Basic evidence clearly indicate that RAS blockade exerts potent antiatherosclerotic effects, not only reducing blood pressure, but also through the anti-inflammatory, antiproliferative, and antioxidant effects [80]. At this regard, it has been reported that treatment with the ACE-inhibitor trandolapril reduces endothelial dysfunction in hyperlipidemic rabbits [13]. In addition, administration of quinapril reduced macrophage infiltration in atherosclerotic lesions in femoral arteries in rabbits through the direct inhibition of macrophage chemoattractant protein (MCP)-1 expression. There is a large consensus that the anti-atherosclerotic properties of both ACE-inhibitors and ARBs are independent from of blood pressure reduction, since the use of other antihypertensive drugs did not produce similar actions. However, the favourable effects of the RAS blockade have been also reported in animal models of hypertension. In particular, in stroke prone spontaneously hypertensive rats (SHR-SP) administration of ramipril reduced mortality and improved left-ventricular hypertrophy, cardiac and endothelial functions [56],indicating that ACE inhibitors reduce cardiovascular risk and atherosclerosis in animal model of essential hypertension. These pharmacological effects in SHR-SP rats were documented also for ARBs as losartan [99], and telmisartan [96].

RAS Inhibition and CV Events

Stroke

Clinical Evidence: The Ang II plays an important role in brain circulation, homeostasis and stroke prevention, both of which are mediated through its receptors AT_1, AT_2, and may be AT_4. The stroke-protective effects of ARBs are mediated through their dual action of blocking the AT_1 receptors and at the same time of allowing Ang II to stimulate the AT_2 and AT_4 receptors, leading to local cerebral vasodilatation and an increase in cerebral blood flow [14]. The favorable effect of RAS inhibition on incidence of stroke in hypertensive patients is well documented. However, it is still debated whether ARBs are more effective than ACE-inhibitors in the prevention of stroke. The first meta-analysis was published by Turnbull et al. in 2003 [97]. They analyzed 29 trials (162,341 participants). Their analysis showed that ACE-inhibitors-based treatment reduced the risk of stroke compared with placebo by 28 %; and ARBs-based treatment reduced the risk of stroke compared with control regimens by 21 %. In 2008 Reboldi et al. [70] analyzed six trials and included 31,632 patients randomized to ARBs and 18,292 patients randomized to ACE-inhibitors. This analysis showed that administration of ARBs was associated with a small but statistically significant reduction in the risk of stroke compared with administration of ACE-inhibitors. This last meta-analysis seems to indicate that compared with ACE-inhibitors, ARBs have a slightly greater protective effect on stroke. However, in 2009 it was published an other meta-analysis [58] that showed no difference in terms of neuro-protection between ACE-inhibitors and ARBs. This analysis considered 20 randomized, controlled trials (108,286 patients), demonstrated benefit of ARBs on the risk of stroke when compared with placebo. However, was no evidence of the benefit when comparing ARBs with ACE-inhibitors was reported.

Experimental evidence: At experimental level, there are some evidence indicating that ARBs compared to ACE-inhibitors might have a greater and specific cerebral protective effect. In fact, many animal studies in gerbils and rats have shown that ARBs decrease the volume and the extent of infracted brain tissue after induction of acute cerebral ischemia by carotid ligation or middle cerebral artery occlusion (MCAO). For example, The mortality of gerbils after induction of acute brain ischemia by ligation of the right carotid artery was significantly decreased with pretreatment with the selective AT1 receptor blocker losartan or the selective AT2 receptor agonist PD 123319, but not with the ACE inhibitor enalapril [22]. Moreover, the neurological outcome following induction of cerebral ischemia in the rat was improved by intracerebral administration of low doses of the ARB irbesartan, and such effect was prevented by the co-administration of an AT2 receptor blocker [53]. In Wistar rats pretreatment with low doses of candesartan (0.1 mg/kg body weight, twice daily) and ramipril (0.01 mg/kg body weight, twice daily) did not reduce blood pressure during MCAO, whereas ramipril high dose (0.1 mg/kg body weight, twice daily) did. However, candesartan, but not ramipril at any dose, significantly reduced stroke volume and improved neurological outcome. Poststroke mRNA and protein of the neurotrophin receptor, TrkB, were significantly elevated in animals treated with candesartan, but not ramipril, suggesting that RAS-blockade by candesartan, but not ramipril exerts a neuroprotective action after focal ischemia [47]. Together, these experiments allow to hypothesize that Ang II exerts its cerebroprotective effects via stimulation of the AT2 receptors, and this action is further enhanced with selective blockade of the AT1 receptors. In this case, upon the distribution (brain, heart) AT_2 receptors play a different physiological role.

Myocardial Infarction

Clinical Evidence: The effect of RAS inhibition on incidence of myocardial infarction is still debated. This controversy started from the publication of results of VALUE [40], in which, in hypertensive patients, there was detected a significant increase of myocardial infarction in the Valsartan group compared with the Amlodipine group. Following this study, it was been hypothesized that ARBs rather than to be protective against myocardial ischemia increased the risk of myocardial infarction. This hypothesis was corroborated by several interventional studies, in particular the CHARM-alternative Trial showed a significant 36 % increase in myocardial infarction with candesartan (versus placebo) despite a reduction in BP (4.4 and 3.9 mmHg for systolic diastolic, respectively; vs placebo treatment) [26]; furthermore, in the LIFE study the

ARB losartan did not reduce rates of myocardial infarction despite a 1.7 mmHg lower pulse pressure compared with atenolol [17]. On the basis of these evidence Verma and Strauss raised the hypothesis that ARBs, unlike ACE inhibitors, rather to be protective, were either neutral or increase the rates of myocardial infarction despite their beneficial effects on reducing blood pressure [101]. This theory, called "ARB-myocardial infarction paradox" was not confirmed by the meta-analysis published by Bangalore et al. These authors analyzed 37 trials which randomised 147,020 participants, 73,298 (49.8 %) to ARBs and 73,722 (50.2 %) to controls. The average follow-up was 3.3 years (range 1–6.5 years). ARBs were not associated with any increase in the risk of myocardial infarction when compared with controls (relative risk 0.99, 95 % confidence interval 0.92–1.07; P=0.85). These results were similar when ARBs were compared with either placebo or with active treatment. These authors concluded that ARBs do not increase the risk of myocardial infarction; however, they do not have beneficial effect for the outcome of myocardial infarction or cardiovascular mortality. However, further meta-analyses showed opposite results. In particular, Stauss and Hall [92] analyzed 11 trials (55,050 patients). In details, five trials compared ARBs versus ACE inhibitors, four trials compared ARBs and placebo, and two trials compared ARBs versus non-ACE inhibitors. The main result of this analysis showed a rates of global death of 14.0 %; CV death of 9.2 %; non-CV death of 4.7 %; stroke of 4.4 %; and myocardial infarction of 6.3 %. Only incidence of stroke was lower in patients treated with ARBs compared with placebo. Global death was not reduced by ARBs whereas myocardial infarction was significantly increased by 8 %. The results of this meta-analysis clearly demonstrate that compared with placebo, ACE inhibitors reduce the incidence of myocardial infarction and CV death, whereas there is no evidence than an ARBs are better than placebo.

Experimental evidence: The results of these analyses clearly indicate that ACE inhibitors and ARBs acts through different mechanisms of action. In particular, the inhibition of breakdown of bradykinin exerted by ACE inhibitors represents an 'adjunctive' favorable mechanism. Bradykinin inhibits both platelet aggregation and circulating PAI-I levels and is one of the most potent stimulators of tissue plasminogen activator. Furthermore, bradykinin promotes vasodilatation via the release of prostacyclin, NO, and endothelium-derived hyperpolarizing factor. Long-term treatment with ACEIs augments both bradykinin-induced peripheral vasodilatation and the release of tissue plasminogen activator to levels that approximate those seen during systemic thrombolytic therapy. On the other hand, bradikinin is also a mediator of ischemic preconditioning which is a physiological phenomenon in which non-sustained, repetitive, sub-lethal ischemic stimulation enhances tolerance to a subsequent prolonged ischemic stress. Preconditioning has great pathophysiological relevance, since it confers protection against ischemia-induced cell death to those organs that are composed of terminally differentiated cells, like the brain and heart. In addition, we have recently demonstrated, in endothelial cells, that precondition stimulates the release of bradikinin, which in turn, through a autocrine-paracrine mechanism activates cell survival pathways.

Experimental evidence indicate that AT_2 receptor stimulation, rather than to be beneficial, as previously proposed, is detrimental for cardiovascular system. In particular, it has been described that under certain circumstances stimulation of AT_2 receptors promotes fibrosis, and hypertrophy, as well as pro-atherogenic and pro-inflammatory effects. In transgenic mice, the chronic overexpression of AT_2 induces Ca^{2+}- and pH-dependent contractile dysfunction in ventricular myocytes, as well as loss of the inotropic response to Ang II [63]. AT_2-deficient mice are protected against cardiac hypertrophy [83], whereas overexpression of AT_2 in human cardiac myocytes is associated with increased cardiac hypertrophy [16]. In addition, a critical role for an AT_2 receptor in mediating dilated cardiomyopathy and cardiac hypertrophy has been demonstrated [33]. Furthermore it has been documented that AT_2 receptors inhibit vascular endothelial growth factor–induced angiogenesis in endothelial cells [8]. Finally, evidence in human myocytes suggests that Ang II may promote plaque rupture by augmenting matrix metalloproteinase-1 in an AT_2-dependent fashion and by preventing growth of vascular smooth muscle cells with reduced collagen deposition and additional cellular apoptosis within advanced plaques [43].

Therefore, at molecular level, ACE inhibitors exert their favorable action on cardiovascular morbidity and mortality by increasing cardiac cell protection, and this effect is not shared by ARBs.

RAS Inhibitors and Mortality

The effects of inhibition of RAS obtained with either ACE-inhibitors or ARBs on all-cause mortality in hypertensive patients is have been evaluated by van Vark and colleagues. They, showed, in a recent meta-analysis that considered 20 randomized studies, included 158,998 patients (71,401 RAS inhibitor; 87,597 control) followed for 4.3 years, that RAS inhibition reduced by 5 % all-cause mortality (HR: 0.95, 95 % CI: 0.91–1.00, P=0.032), and by 7 % cardiovascular mortality (HR: 0.93, 95 % CI: 0.88–0.99, P=0.018). However, when the effects of ACE-inhibitors and ARBs were analyzed separately, ACE inhibitors were associated with a statistically significant 10 % reduction in all-cause mortality, while no mortality reduction was demonstrated for ARBs treatment. Therefore, it is reasonable to speculate that reduction of all-cause mortality recorded in the analyzed cohort was entirely driven by the favorable effects of the ACE-inhibitors. The results of this analysis seem to be consistent with other meta-analysis which confirm that ACE-inhibitors, but not ARBs, are able to reduce cardiovascular morbidity and mortality. The goal of hypertension management must be the reduction of global CV risk. Recent evidence from clinical trials and meta-analyses show that treatment with ACE inhibitors, but not with ARBs, leads to a statistically significant further reduction in mortality in hypertensive patients [76]. This provide a convincing evidence that ACE inhibitors should be considered the drugs of first choice and ARBs should be restricted to patients intolerant of ACE inhibitors.

References

1. Abuissa H, Jones PG, Marso SP, et al. Angiotensin-converting enzyme inhibitors or angiotensin receptor blockers for prevention of type 2 diabetes: a meta-analysis of randomized clinical trials. J Am Coll Cardiol. 2005;46(5):821–6.
2. Ailhaud G. Cross talk between adipocytes and their precursors: relationships with adipose tissue development and blood pressure. Ann N Y Acad Sci. 1999;892:127–33.
3. Andersson P, Cederholm T, Johansson AS, et al. Captopril-impaired production of tumor necrosis factor-alpha-induced interleukin-1beta in human monocytes is associated with altered intracellular distribution of nuclear factor-kappaB. J Lab Clin Med. 2002;140(2):103–9.
4. Arbin V, Claperon N, Fournie-Zaluski MC, et al. Acute effect of the dual angiotensin-converting enzyme and neutral endopeptidase 24–11 inhibitor mixanpril on insulin sensitivity in obese Zucker rat. Br J Pharmacol. 2001;133(4):495–502.
5. Baguet JP, Asmar R, Valensi P, et al. Effects of candesartan cilexetil on carotid remodeling in hypertensive diabetic patients: the MITEC study. Vasc Health Risk Manag. 2009;5(1):175–83.
6. Bähr IN, Tretter P, Krüger J, et al. High-dose treatment with telmisartan induces monocytic peroxisome proliferator-activated receptor-γ target genes in patients with the metabolic syndrome. Hypertension. 2011;58(4):725–32.
7. Bendall JK, Cave AC, Heymes C, et al. Pivotal role of a gp91(phox)-containing NADPH oxidase in angiotensin II-induced cardiac hypertrophy in mice. Circulation. 2002;105(3):293–6.
8. Benndorf R, Böger RH, Ergün S, et al. Angiotensin II type 2 receptor inhibits vascular endothelial growth factor-induced migration and in vitro tube formation of human endothelial cells. Circ Res. 2003;93(5):438–47.
9. Bruckschlegel G, Holmer SR, Jandeleit K, et al. Blockade of the renin-angiotensin system in cardiac pressure-overload hypertrophy in rats. Hypertension. 1995;25(2):250–9.
10. Carlsson PO, Berne C, Jansson L. Angiotensin II and the endocrine pancreas: effects on islet blood flow and insulin secretion in rats. Diabetologia. 1998;41(2):127–33.

11. Carvalho CR, Thirone AC, Gontijo JA, et al. Effect of captopril, losartan, and bradykinin on early steps of insulin action. Diabetes. 1997;46(12):1950–7.
12. Catapano F, Chiodini P, De Nicola L, et al. Antiproteinuric response to dual blockade of the renin-angiotensin system in primary glomerulonephritis: meta-analysis and metaregression. Am J Kidney Dis. 2008;52(3):475–85.
13. Chobanian AV, Haudenschild CC, Nickerson C, et al. Trandolapril inhibits atherosclerosis in the Watanabe heritable hyperlipidemic rabbit. Hypertension. 1992;20(4):473–7.
14. Chrysant SG. The role of angiotensin II receptors in stroke protection. Curr Hypertens Rep. 2012;14(3):202–8.
15. Conlin PR, Spence JD, Williams B, et al. Angiotensin II antagonists for hypertension: are there differences in efficacy? Am J Hypertens. 2000;13(4 Pt 1):418–26.
16. D'Amore A, Black MJ, Thomas WG. The angiotensin II type 2 receptor causes constitutive growth of cardiomyocytes and does not antagonize angiotensin II type 1 receptor-mediated hypertrophy. Hypertension. 2005;46(6):1347–54.
17. Dahlöf B, Devereux RB, Kjeldsen SE, et al. Cardiovascular morbidity and mortality in the Losartan Intervention For Endpoint reduction in hypertension study (LIFE): a randomised trial against atenolol. Lancet. 2002;359(9311):995–1003.
18. Dal Ponte DB, Fogt DL, Jacob S, et al. Interactions of captopril and verapamil on glucose tolerance and insulin action in an animal model of insulin resistance. Metabolism. 1998;47(8):982–7.
19. Daugherty A, Rateri DL, Lu H, et al. Hypercholesterolemia stimulates angiotensin peptide synthesis and contributes to atherosclerosis through the AT1A receptor. Circulation. 2004;110(25):3849–57.
20. Engeli S, Sharma AM. Role of adipose tissue for cardiovascular-renal regulation in health and disease. Horm Metab Res. 2000;32(11–12):485–99.
21. Fagard RH, Celis H, Thijs L, et al. Regression of left ventricular mass by antihypertensive treatment: a meta-analysis of randomized comparative studies. Hypertension. 2009;54(5):1084–91.
22. Fernandez LA, Caride VJ, Strömberg C, et al. Angiotensin AT2 receptor stimulation increases survival in gerbils with abrupt unilateral carotid ligation. J Cardiovasc Pharmacol. 1994;24(6):937–40.

23. Ferrario CM, Strawn WB. Targeting the RAAS for the treatment of atherosclerosis. Drug Discov Today Ther Strat. 2005; 2(3):221–9.

24. Fryer LG, Hajduch E, Rencurel F, et al. Activation of glucose transport by AMP-activated protein kinase via stimulation of nitric oxide synthase. Diabetes. 2000;49(12):1978–85.

25. Gorzelniak K, Engeli S, Janke J, et al. Hormonal regulation of the human adipose-tissue renin-angiotensin system: relationship to obesity and hypertension. J Hypertens. 2002;20(5):965–73.

26. Granger CB, McMurray JJ, Yusuf S, et al. Effects of candesartan in patients with chronic heart failure and reduced left-ventricular systolic function intolerant to angiotensin-converting-enzyme inhibitors: the CHARM-Alternative trial. Lancet. 2003; 362(9386):772–6.

27. Grassi G, Seravalle G, Dell'Oro R, et al. Comparative effects of candesartan and hydrochlorothiazide on blood pressure, insulin sensitivity, and sympathetic drive in obese hypertensive individuals: results of the CROSS study. J Hypertens. 2003;21(9):1761–9.

28. Gruppo Italiano di Studi Epidemiologici in Nefrologia. Randomised placebo-controlled trial of effect of ramipril on decline in glomerular filtration rate and risk of terminal renal failure in proteinuric, non-diabetic nephropathy. Lancet. 1997;349(9069):1857–63.

29. Hansson L, Lindholm LH, Ekbom T, et al. Randomised trial of old and new antihypertensive drugs in elderly patients: cardiovascular mortality and morbidity the Swedish Trial in Old Patients with Hypertension-2 study. Lancet. 1999;354(9192):1751–6.

30. Hansson L, Lindholm LH, Niskanen L, et al. Effect of angiotensin-converting-enzyme inhibition compared with conventional therapy on cardiovascular morbidity and mortality in hypertension: the Captopril Prevention Project (CAPPP) randomised trial. Lancet. 1999;353(9153):611–6.

31. Henriksen EJ, Jacob S. Effects of captopril on glucose transport activity in skeletal muscle of obese Zucker rats. Metabolism. 1995;44(2):267–72.

32. Hirohata A, Yamamoto K, Miyoshi T, et al. Impact of olmesartan on progression of coronary atherosclerosis a serial volumetric intravascular ultrasound analysis from the OLIVUS (impact of OLmesarten on progression of coronary atherosclerosis: evaluation by intravascular ultrasound) trial. J Am Coll Cardiol. 2010;55(10):976–82.

33. Ichihara S, Senbonmatsu T, Price Jr E, et al. Angiotensin II type 2 receptor is essential for left ventricular hypertrophy and cardiac fibrosis in chronic angiotensin II-induced hypertension. Circulation. 2001;104(3):346–51.

34. Iino Y, Hayashi M, Kawamura T, et al. Renoprotective effect of losartan in comparison to amlodipine in patients with chronic kidney disease and hypertension – a report of the Japanese Losartan Therapy Intended for the Global Renal Protection in Hypertensive Patients (JLIGHT) study. Hypertens Res. 2004;27(1):21–30.

35. ONTARGET Investigators, Yusuf S, Teo KK, et al. Telmisartan, ramipril, or both in patients at high risk for vascular events. N Engl J Med. 2008;358(15):1547–59.

36. Jacob S, Henriksen EJ, Fogt DL, et al. Effects of trandolapril and verapamil on glucose transport in insulin-resistant rat skeletal muscle. Metabolism. 1996;45(5):535–41.

37. Jafar TH, Schmid CH, Landa M, et al. Angiotensin-converting enzyme inhibitors and progression of nondiabetic renal disease. A meta-analysis of patient-level data. Ann Intern Med. 2001;135(2):73–87.

38. Jafar TH, Stark PC, Schmid CH, et al. Proteinuria as a modifiable risk factor for the progression of non-diabetic renal disease. Kidney Int. 2001;60(3):1131–40.

39. Jones BH, Standridge MK, Taylor JW, et al. Angiotensinogen gene expression in adipose tissue: analysis of obese models and hormonal and nutritional control. Am J Physiol. 1997;273(1 Pt 2):R236–42.

40. Julius S, Kjeldsen SE, Weber M, et al. Outcomes in hypertensive patients at high cardiovascular risk treated with regimens based on valsartan or amlodipine: the VALUE randomised trial. Lancet. 2004;363(9426):2022–31.

41. Kanome T, Watanabe T, Nishio K, et al. Angiotensin II upregulates acyl-CoA: cholesterol acyltransferase-1 via the angiotensin II Type 1 receptor in human monocyte-macrophages. Hypertens Res. 2008;31(9):1801–10.

42. Keidar S, Kaplan M, Hoffman A, et al. Angiotensin II stimulates macrophage-mediated oxidation of low density lipoproteins. Atherosclerosis. 1995;115(2):201–15.

43. Kim MP, Zhou M, Wahl LM. Angiotensin II increases human monocyte matrix metalloproteinase-1 through the AT2 receptor and prostaglandin E2: implications for atherosclerotic plaque rupture. J Leukoc Biol. 2005;78(1):195–201.

44. Klingbeil AU, Schneider M, Martus P, et al. A meta-analysis of the effects of treatment on left ventricular mass in essential hypertension. Am J Med. 2003;115(1):41–6.
45. Koh KK, Han SH, Chung WJ, et al. Comparison of effects of losartan, irbesartan, and candesartan on flow-mediated brachial artery dilation and on inflammatory and thrombolytic markers in patients with systemic hypertension. Am J Cardiol. 2004;93(11):1432–5, A10.
46. Kojima M, Shiojima I, Yamazaki T, et al. Angiotensin II receptor antagonist TCV-116 induces regression of hypertensive left ventricular hypertrophy in vivo and inhibits the intracellular signaling pathway of stretch-mediated cardiomyocyte hypertrophy in vitro. Circulation. 1994;89(5):2204–11.
47. Krikov M, Thone-Reineke C, Müller S, et al. Candesartan but not ramipril pretreatment improves outcome after stroke and stimulates neurotrophin BNDF/TrkB system in rats. J Hypertens. 2008;26(3):544–52.
48. Kshirsagar AV, Joy MS, Hogan SL, et al. Effect of ACE inhibitors in diabetic and nondiabetic chronic renal disease: a systematic overview of randomized placebo-controlled trials. Am J Kidney Dis. 2000;35(4):695–707.
49. Kunz R, Friedrich C, Wolbers M, et al. Meta-analysis: effect of monotherapy and combination therapy with inhibitors of the renin angiotensin system on proteinuria in renal disease. Ann Intern Med. 2008;148(1):30–48.
50. Kyvelou SM, Vyssoulis GP, Karpanou EA, et al. Effects of antihypertensive treatment with angiotensin II receptor blockers on lipid profile: an open multi-drug comparison trial. Hellenic J Cardiol. 2006;47(1):21–8.
51. Lau DC, Dhillon B, Yan H, et al. Adipokines: molecular links between obesity and atheroslcerosis. Am J Physiol Heart Circ Physiol. 2005;288(5):H2031–41.
52. Lewington S, Clarke R, Qizilbash N, et al. Age-specific relevance of usual blood pressure to vascular mortality: a meta-analysis of individual data for one million adults in 61 prospective studies. Lancet. 2002;360(9349):1903–13.
53. Li J, Culman J, Hörtnagl H, et al. Angiotensin AT2 receptor protects against cerebral ischemia-induced neuronal injury. FASEB J. 2005;19(6):617–9.
54. Li D, Saldeen T, Romeo F, et al. Oxidized LDL upregulates angiotensin II type 1 receptor expression in cultured human coronary

artery endothelial cells: the potential role of transcription factor NF-kappaB. Circulation. 2000;102(16):1970–6.

55. Lindholm LH, Persson M, Alaupovic P, et al. Metabolic outcome during 1 year in newly detected hypertensives: results of the Antihypertensive Treatment and Lipid Profile in a North of Sweden Efficacy Evaluation (ALPINE study). J Hypertens. 2003;21(8):1563–74.

56. Linz W, Jessen T, Becker RH, et al. Long-term ACE inhibition doubles lifespan of hypertensive rats. Circulation. 1997; 96(9):3164–72.

57. Lonn E, Yusuf S, Dzavik V, et al. Effects of ramipril and vitamin E on atherosclerosis: the study to evaluate carotid ultrasound changes in patients treated with ramipril and vitamin E (SECURE). Circulation. 2001;103(7):919–25.

58. Lu GC, Cheng JW, Zhu KM, et al. A systematic review of angio-tensin receptor blockers in preventing stroke. Stroke. 2009;40(12):3876–8.

59. Mancia G, Fagard R, Narkiewicz K, et al. 2013 ESH/ESC guide-lines for the management of arterial hypertension: the Task Force for the Management of Arterial Hypertension of the European Society of Hypertension (ESH) and of the European Society of Cardiology (ESC). Eur Heart J. 2013;34(28):2159–219.

60. Martinez-Martin FJ, Rodriguez-Rosas H, Peiro-Martinez I, et al. Olmesartan/amlodipine vs olmesartan/hydrochlorothiazide in hypertensive patients with metabolic syndrome: the OLAS study. J Hum Hypertens. 2011;25(6):346–53.

61. Morel Y, Gadient A, Keller U, et al. Insulin sensitivity in obese hypertensive dyslipidemic patients treated with enalapril or atenolol. J Cardiovasc Pharmacol. 1995;26(2):306–11.

62. Nakao N, Yoshimura A, Morita H, et al. Combination treatment of angiotensin-II receptor blocker and angiotensin-converting-enzyme inhibitor in non-diabetic renal disease (COOPERATE): a randomised controlled trial. Lancet. 2003;361(9352):117–24.

63. Nakayama M, Yan X, Price RL, et al. Chronic ventricular myocyte-specific overexpression of angiotensin II type 2 recep-tor results in intrinsic myocyte contractile dysfunction. Am J Physiol Heart Circ Physiol. 2005;288(1):H317–27.

64. Nickenig G, Sachinidis A, Michaelsen F, et al. Upregulation of vascular angiotensin II receptor gene expression by low-density lipoprotein in vascular smooth muscle cells. Circulation. 1997;95(2):473–8.

65. Nishida Y, Takahashi Y, Nakayama T, et al. Effect of candesartan monotherapy on lipid metabolism in patients with hypertension: a retrospective longitudinal survey using data from electronic medical records. Cardiovasc Diabetol. 2010;9:38.
66. Olsen MH, Wachtell K, Beevers G, et al. Effects of losartan compared with atenolol on lipids in patients with hypertension and left ventricular hypertrophy: the Losartan Intervention For Endpoint reduction in hypertension study. Effects of losartan compared with atenolol on lipids in patients with hypertension and left ventricular hypertrophy: the Losartan Intervention For Endpoint reduction in hypertension study. J Hypertens. 2009;27(3):567–74.
67. Parhofer KG, Münzel F, Krekler M. Effect of the angiotensin receptor blocker irbesartan on metabolic parameters in clinical practice: the DO-IT prospective observational study. Cardiovasc Diabetol. 2007;6:36.
68. Pollare T, Lithell H, Berne C. A comparison of the effects of hydrochlorothiazide and captopril on glucose and lipid metabolism in patients with hypertension. N Engl J Med. 1998;321(13):868–73.
69. Putnam K, Shoemaker R, Yiannikouris F, et al. The renin-angiotensin system: a target of and contributor to dyslipidemias, altered glucose homeostasis, and hypertension of the metabolic syndrome. Am J Physiol Heart Circ Physiol. 2012;302(6):H1219–30.
70. Reboldi G, Angeli F, Cavallini C, et al. Comparison between angiotensin-converting enzyme inhibitors and angiotensin receptor blockers on the risk of myocardial infarction, stroke and death: a meta-analysis. J Hypertens. 2008;26(7):1282–9.
71. Reisin E, Weir MR, Falkner B, et al. Lisinopril versus hydrochlorothiazide in obese hypertensive patients: a multicenter placebo-controlled trial. Treatment in Obese Patients With Hypertension (TROPHY) Study Group. Hypertension. 1997;30(1 Pt 1):140–5.
72. Rett K, Wicklmayr M, Dietze GJ, et al. Insulin-induced glucose transporter (GLUT1 and GLUT4) translocation in cardiac muscle tissue is mimicked by bradykinin. Diabetes. 1996;45 Suppl 1:S66–9.
73. Rosei EA, Rizzoni D, Muiesan ML, et al. Effects of candesartan cilexetil and enalapril on inflammatory markers of atherosclerosis in hypertensive patients with non-insulin-dependent diabetes mellitus. J Hypertens. 2005;23(2):435–44.
74. Rotimi C, Cooper R, Ogunbiyi O, et al. Hypertension, serum angiotensinogen, and molecular variants of the angiotensinogen gene among Nigerians. Circulation. 1997;95(10):2348–50.

75. Ruiz-Ortega M, Lorenzo O, Suzuki Y, et al. Proinflammatory actions of angiotensins. Curr Opin Nephrol Hypertens. 2001;10(3):321–9.
76. Ruschitzka F, Taddei S. Angiotensin-converting enzyme inhibitors: first-line agents in cardiovascular protection? Eur Heart J. 2012;33(16):1996–8.
77. Sadoshima J, Izumo S. Molecular characterization of angiotensin II – induced hypertrophy of cardiac myocytes and hyperplasia of cardiac fibroblasts. Critical role of the AT1 receptor subtype. Circ Res. 1993;73(3):413–23.
78. Sadoshima J, Izumo S. The cellular and molecular response of cardiac myocytes to mechanical stress. Annu Rev Physiol. 1997;59:551–71.
79. Sadoshima J, Xu Y, Slayter HS, et al. Autocrine release of angiotensin II mediates stretch-induced hypertrophy of cardiac myocytes in vitro. Cell. 1993;75(5):977–84.
80. Schmieder RE, Hilgers KF, Schlaich MP, et al. Renin-angiotensin system and cardiovascular risk. Lancet. 2007;369(9568):1208–19.
81. Schmieder RE, Martus P, Klingbeil A. Reversal of left ventricular hypertrophy in essential hypertension. A meta-analysis of randomized double-blind studies. JAMA. 1996;275(19): 1507–13.
82. Schupp M, Janke J, Clasen R, et al. Angiotensin type 1 receptor blockers induce peroxisome proliferator-activated receptor-gamma activity. Circulation. 2004;109(17):2054–7.
83. Senbonmatsu T, Ichihara S, Price Jr E, et al. Evidence for angiotensin II type 2 receptor-mediated cardiac myocyte enlargement during in vivo pressure overload. J Clin Invest. 2000;106(3):R25–9.
84. Sharma AM, Janke J, Gorzelniak K, et al. Angiotensin blockade prevents type 2 diabetes by formation of fat cells. Hypertension. 2002;40(5):609–11.
85. Shiuchi T, Cui TX, Wu L, et al. ACE inhibitor improves insulin resistance in diabetic mouse via bradykinin and NO. Hypertension. 2002;40(3):329–34.
86. Shyu KG, Chen JJ, Shih NL, et al. Angiotensinogen gene expression is induced by cyclical mechanical stretch in cultured rat cardiomyocytes. Biochem Biophys Res Commun. 1995;211(1):241–8.
87. Sola S, Mir MQ, Cheema FA, et al. Irbesartan and lipoic acid improve endothelial function and reduce markers of inflammation in the metabolic syndrome: results of the Irbesartan

and Lipoic Acid in Endothelial Dysfunction (ISLAND) study. Circulation. 2005;111(3):343–8.

88. Sonoda M, Aoyagi T, Takenaka K, et al. A one-year study of the antiatherosclerotic effect of the angiotensin-II receptor blocker losartan in hypertensive patients. A comparison with angiotension-converting enzyme inhibitors. Int Heart J. 2008;49(1):95–103.

89. Steen MS, Foianini KR, Youngblood EB, et al. Interactions of exercise training and ACE inhibition on insulin action in obese Zucker rats. J Appl Physiol. 1999;86(6):2044–51.

90. Stenvinkel P, Andersson P, Wang T, et al. Do ACE-inhibitors suppress tumour necrosis factor-alpha production in advanced chronic renal failure? J Intern Med. 1999;246(5):503–7.

91. Stenvinkel P, Ketteler M, Johnson RJ, et al. IL-10, IL-6, and TNF-alpha: central factors in the altered cytokine network of uremia – the good, the bad, and the ugly. Kidney Int. 2005;67(4):1216–33.

92. Strauss MH, Hall AS. Angiotensin receptor blockers may increase risk of myocardial infarction: unraveling the ARB-MI paradox. Circulation. 2006;114(8):838–54.

93. Suzuki J, Matsubara H, Urakami M, et al. Rat angiotensin II (type 1A) receptor mRNA regulation and subtype expression in myocardial growth and hypertrophy. Circ Res. 1993;73(3):439–47.

94. Suzuki Y, Ruiz-Ortega M, Gomez-Guerrero C, et al. Angiotensin II, the immune system and renal diseases: another road for RAS? Nephrol Dial Transplant. 2003;18(8):1423–6.

95. Taal MW, Brenner BM. Renoprotective benefits of RAS inhibition: from ACEI to angiotensin II antagonists. Kidney Int. 2000;57(5):1803–17.

96. Thoene-Reineke C, Rumschüssel K, Schmerbach K, et al. Prevention and intervention studies with telmisartan, ramipril and their combination in different rat stroke models. PLoS One. 2011;6(8):e23646. doi:10.1371/journal.pone.0023646.

97. Turnbull F, Blood Pressure Lowering Treatment Trialists' Collaboration. Effects of different blood-pressure-lowering regimens on major cardiovascular events: results of prospectively-designed overviews of randomised trials. Lancet. 2003;362(9395):1527–35.

98. Uehara M, Kishikawa H, Isami S, et al. Effect on insulin sensitivity of angiotensin converting enzyme inhibitors with or without a sulphydryl group: bradykinin may improve insulin resistance in dogs and humans. Diabetologia. 1994;37(3):300–7.

99. Vacher E, Richer C, Giudicelli JF. Effects of losartan on cerebral arteries in stroke-prone spontaneously hypertensive rats. J Hypertens. 1996;14(11):1341–8.

100. Vasan RS, Larson MG, Leip EP, et al. Impact of high-normal blood pressure on the risk of cardiovascular disease. N Engl J Med. 2001;345(18):1291–7.

101. Verma S, Strauss M. Angiotensin receptor blockers and myocardial infarction. BMJ. 2004;329(7477):1248–9.

102. Vogt L, Navis G, Köster J, et al. The angiotensin II receptor antagonist telmisartan reduces urinary albumin excretion in patients with isolated systolic hypertension: results of a randomized, double-blind, placebo-controlled trial. J Hypertens. 2005;23(11):2055–61.

103. Weinberg EO, Schoen FJ, George D, et al. Angiotensin-converting enzyme inhibition prolongs survival and modifies the transition to heart failure in rats with pressure overload hypertrophy due to ascending aortic stenosis. Circulation. 1994;90(3):1410–22.

104. Yamazaki T, Komuro I, Kudoh S, et al. Angiotensin II partly mediates mechanical stress-induced cardiac hypertrophy. Circ Res. 1995;77(2):258–65.

105. Yusuf S, Sleight P, Pogue J, et al. Effects of an angiotensin-converting-enzyme inhibitor, ramipril, on cardiovascular events in high-risk patients. The Heart Outcomes Prevention Evaluation Study Investigators. N Engl J Med. 2000;342(3):145–53.

Chapter 2
ACE Inhibitor and Renin–Angiotensin System the Cornerstone of Therapy for Systolic Heart Failure

Claudio Borghi, Filippo Del Corso, Simone Faenza, and Eugenio Cosentino

Definition of Heart Failure

Heart failure (HF) can be defined as an abnormality of cardiac structure or function leading to failure of the heart to deliver oxygen at a rate commensurate with the requirements of the metabolizing tissues, despite normal filling pressures (or only at the expense of increased filling pressures) [1]. HF can be also defined, clinically, as a syndrome in which patients have typical symptoms (e.g. breathlessness, ankle swelling, and fatigue) and signs (e.g. elevated jugular venous pressure, pulmonary crackles, and displaced apex beat) resulting from an abnormality of cardiac structure or function. The diagnosis of HF, according to the guidelines of the European Society of

C. Borghi (✉)
Cattedra di Medicina Interna, Ospedale S.Orsola.Malpighi,
Via Albertoni 15, Bologna 40138, Italy

Department of Medicine, University of Bologna, Bologna, Italy
e-mail: claudio.borghi@unibo.it

F. Del Corso • S. Faenza • E. Cosentino
Department of Medicine, University of Bologna, Bologna, Italy

© Springer International Publishing Switzerland 2015   41
P. Perrone Filardi (ed.), *ACEi and ARBS in Hypertension and Heart Failure*, Current Cardiovascular Therapy 5,
DOI 10.1007/978-3-319-09788-6_2

Cardiology, can be difficult and is based on a criterion of clinical evaluation, which relies on the clinical history, physical examination and appropriate investigations [2]. For this reason is more important the need to obtain objective evidence of a structural or functional cardiac abnormality that is thought to account for the patient's symptoms and signs, to secure the diagnosis of HF.

From the point of view of the classification HF is divided into acute and chronic form. The chronic form is the most common form of HF and its clinical feature most obvious are certainly frequent exacerbations evolution sometimes to acute complications. In this situation the patient may be described as "decompensated" and when a chronic stable HF deteriorates suddenly, i.e. "acutely", usually leading to hospital admission, an event of considerable prognostic importance. In this condition the term of acute HF is used to indicate pathological conditions such as acute pulmonary edema (cardiogenic) and cardiogenic shock, however, very different from the perspective of pathophysiological and clinical. Therefore it would be advisable not to use the term to refer to acute HF in these situations, but it is advisable to choose the most appropriate terms of acute pulmonary edema and cardiogenic shock.

HF can also be classified on the basis of the prevailing characteristics of ventricular dysfunction. In most cases the HF is associated with systolic dysfunction of the left ventricle (LV) that, if determined by echocardiography or other imaging tests (e.g. Cardiac Magnetic Resonance, Single-Photon Emission Computed Tomography) is manifested by a depression of the left ventricular ejection fraction (LVEF). Often in patients with HF is present next to systolic dysfunction also diastolic dysfunction that may be more or less relevant and sometimes presents even in the absence of impaired systolic function. The diagnosis of HF from diastolic dysfunction is formulated based on the presence of symptoms and signs of heart and instrumental to the demonstration of a normal LVEF at rest. Furthermore some patients, particularly those with 'idiopathic' dilated cardiomyopathy, may also show substantial or even complete recovery of LV systolic function with therapy [including an angiotensin-converting enzyme

(ACE) inhibitor, beta-blocker, and mineralocorticoid receptor antagonist (MRA)].

Epidemiology, Incidence, Prevalence and Natural History of Heart Failure

HF is one of the issues most relevant clinical and health in industrialized countries. Infact the HF is the leading cause of hospitalization and is a major cause of disability in patients older than 65 years. Over the past 30 years, the prevalence of cardiovascular diseases has been generally decreasing, while that of HF has been progressively increasing. Approximately 1–2 % of the adult population in developed countries has HF, with the prevalence rising to ≥10 % among persons 70 years of age or older [3].

In industrialized countries, this amount is expected to rise inevitably because of the increase in the average age of the population and in view of the fact that the overall mortality resulting from cardiovascular events is being reduced, while the quod vitam prognosis of patients with HF is, albeit slightly, improved due to the more aggressive treatment.

With regard to the distribution of HF in terms of LV dysfunction that measured by echocardiography between sexes, 51 % of men but only 28 % of women had a LVEF <40 % [4] (Fig. 2.1).

The incidence of HF and its trends are highly variable. The incidence raw (not adjusted for age) in the general population ranges from 1 to 5 cases per 1,000 person-years (28–34), while the data from the largest population-based studies report an incidence ranging from 1 to 2 per 1,000 cases per year. The wide variability in the data of incidence is largely due to the use of diagnostic criteria is not unique and only partially defined. In addition, the incidence data could be made further inaccurate by several factors such as the low percentage of patients autopsied, the economic interest in excluding HF as a discharge diagnosis tab nosographic and the difficulty of framing this syndrome as a primary diagnosis or secondary.

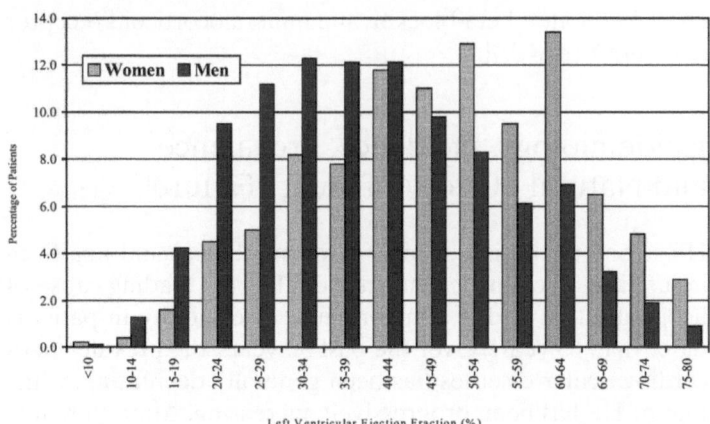

FIG. 2.1 Distribution of left ventricular ejection fraction measured in women and men enrolled in the EuroHeart Failure survey (From Cleland et al. [4])

One datum definitely ascertained is represented by the exponential increase in the incidence of HF with advancing age (Fig. 2.2). With regard to changes in the incidence of HF in time, the Framingham Heart Study showed only a slight decline in incidence during the last three decades, although it must be stated that this study was prior to the use of ACE inhibitors or thrombolytics.

The prevalence of HF is progressively increasing due to the aging of the general population. It is estimated that today the 9.1 % of individuals older than 80 years present a picture of HF and that in the future this percentage is set to grow further. In the United States, it was estimated that in 1997 people aged over 65 years were 33 million (of which about 7.9 million aged greater than or equal to 80 years) and that, by the year 2030, this number will increase to approximately 70 million (of which 18 million aged greater than or equal to 80 years). It may therefore be expected, even with conservative estimates, that, by that time, the number of elderly patients with HF will double, reaching a value of 3.6 million. The prevalence of HF varies from 3 to 20 individuals

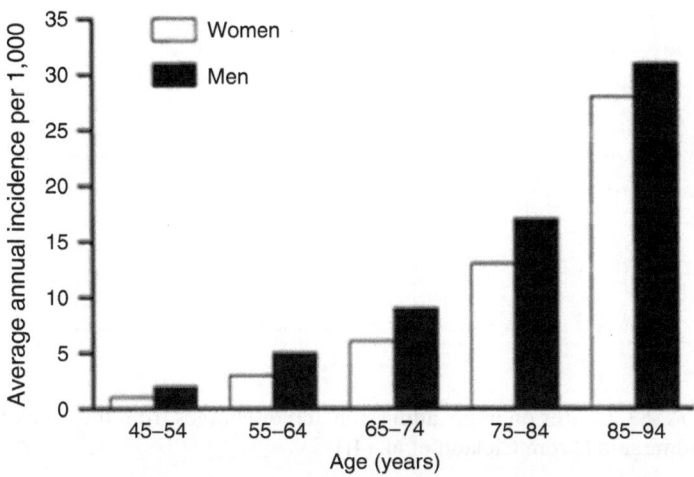

FIG. 2.2 The exponential increase in the incidence of HF with advancing age

per 1,000 people, with higher figures for individuals over the age of 65 years.

Before the modern era of treatment, 60–70 % of patients died within 5 years of diagnosis and 13.5 % died between admission and 12 weeks follow-up (Fig. 2.3). And there was frequent and recurrent admission to hospital: within 12 weeks of discharge, 24 % of patients had been readmitted (Fig. 2.4). Effective treatment has improved both of these outcomes, with a relative reduction in hospitalization in recent years of 30–50 % and smaller but significant decreases in mortality [4–7].

Aetiology of Heart Failure

The most frequent causes of HF are represented by coronary artery disease (CAD is the cause of approximately two-thirds of cases of systolic HF), cardiomyopathy and hypertension (HBP), while valvular heart disease, congenital heart disease

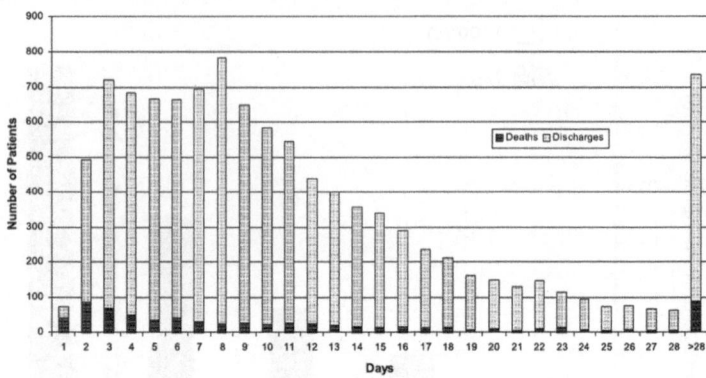

FIG. 2.3 Deaths on index admission and discharges from the time of admission (From Cleland et al. [4])

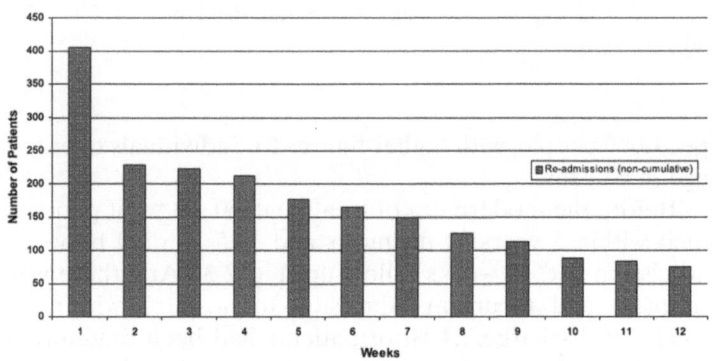

FIG. 2.4 First admission over 12 weeks for any reason from the time of index admission discharge (From Cleland et al. [4])

are more rare (Fig. 2.5). Other causes of systolic HF can be: previous viral infection (recognized or unrecognized), alcohol abuse, hemotherapy (e.g. doxorubicin or trastuzumab), and 'idiopathic' dilated cardiomyopathy (although the cause is thought to be unknown, some of these cases may have a genetic basis) [8]. According to data from the Framingham study HBP, associated or not with ischaemic heart disease, is

Coronary artery disease

Cardiomyopathy:

- **Familial:** hypertrophic; dilated; arrhythmogenic right ventricular cardiomyopathy; restrictive; left ventricular non-compaction;

- **Acquired:** myocarditis (inflammatory cardiomyopathy): infective, immune-mediated, toxic: drugs (e.g. chemotherapy, cocaine), alcohol, heavy metals; endocrine/nutritional; pregnancy; infiltration: amyloidosis, malignancy

Systemic arterial hypertension

Valvular heart disease: mitral; aortic; tricuspid; pulmonary

Congenital heart disease

Pericardial disease: constrictive pericarditis; pericardial effusion

Arrhythmia: Tachyarrhythmia (atrial and ventricular), bradyarrhythmia (sinus node dysfunction)

Conduction disorders: atrioventricular block

High output states: anaemia; sepsis; thyrotoxicosis; Paget's disease; arteriovenous fistula; Beri-beri

Volume overload: renal failure; iatrogenic (e.g. post-operative fluid infusion)

Endocardial disease: endomyocardial diseases with hypereosinophilia [hypereosinophilic syndromes (HES)]; endomyocardial disease without hypereosinophilia [e.g. endomyocardial fibrosis (EMF)]; endocardial fibroelastosis

Fig. 2.5 Causes of HF

the most common cause of HF in the United States. By contrast in Europe, as reported from studies conducted in England and Sweden, the predominant cause of HF is represented by chronic ischaemic heart disease, HBP or cardiomyopathy represent the etiology of HF in percentages lower than 10 %. The data relating to SEOSI, observational epidemiological study conducted in Italy on HF in a population of nearly 4,000 patients referred to hospital centers specialize, identified in the etiology of ischaemic heart disease more frequent with a percentage of 42 % of patients while a role less obvious is found for HBP (20 %), dilated cardiomyopathy (15.3 %) and valvular heart disease (14 %), respectively [9]. Among the plausible reasons for the discrepancies classificative in terms of etiology of HF are certainly numbered the mode of interpretation of the results of epidemiological studies. In particular the role of arterial hypertension is certainly prevalent in all those conditions as the Framingham study in which the development of HF is related to the finding of HBP in each phase of the natural history regardless of the fact that the same has acted as a risk factor for the development of ischaemic heart disease.

In contrast, the role of the same HBP is greatly reduced from those studies (mainly in Europe) in which the development of HF is attributed to the ultimate cause that is responsible for it (e.g., chronic ischaemic heart disease, myocardial infarction [MI] or cardiomyopathy) regardless of the presence anamnestic or clinic HBP.

Pathophysiology of Heart Failure

HF is a complex syndrome with a multifactorial genesis characterized by an inability of the heart to adapt to changes in the metabolic needs of the tissues and supported by hemodynamic changes and different neurohormonal systems, in which the symptoms related to reduced functional capacity and the water retention dominate the clinical picture accompanied with reduced survival. HF can be achieved with alterations in pump function or systolic or diastolic function or filling or, as more often happens, both resulting mainly depression of intrinsic ventricular contractility or changes in mode of contraction. Through the therapeutic restoration of intrinsic contractility of the myocardium can get the simultaneous improvement of systolic function and diastolic function.

Besides the reduction of the intrinsic contractility, a further primary cause of depression of ventricular function can also be the asinergia that makes uneven and asymmetric, and therefore asynchronous, the contraction of the ventricular myocardium for the presence of areas which are contracted little or nothing (zones of hypokinesia and akinesia) or which are contracted with excessive delay (asynchronous areas). The asynchronous contraction of the myocardium, mostly due to ischemic infarction or ventricular arrhythmias, depresses the pump function of the ventricle.

The appearance of alterations of myocardial function affects the development of a series of adaptation mechanisms functional, structural and neurohormonal which are initially able to compensate for the impaired myocardial, but that in a second time can represent elements responsible for a further progression of the disease.

In the initial phase of HF, all conditions characterized by an impaired intrinsic contractility (or inotropism), by distensibility (compliance), by the synergy of contraction of the ventricular walls, by an excessive hemodynamic load or by the association of some of these conditions, induce the heart to resort to various compensatory mechanisms of adaptation, immediate or delayed, aimed to preserve its pump function.

If the overload systolic or diastolic are not removed, the phase of functional insufficiency follows a second phase of re-structural adaptation, characterized by a stimulation of the synthesis of myocytes, resulting in hypertrophy (and according to some authors, also hyperplasia) of the muscle cells and hyperplasia of interstitial component, mainly fibroblasts and matrix collagen. The wall stress also causes a stimulus to gene expression involving oncogenes, myocardial protein (ANP, BNP, angiotensin II). The combination of these processes conditions the development of a parietal hypertrophy. In the terminal stages of HF the maladaptive changes occurring in surviving myocytes and extracellular matrix after myocardial injury (e.g. MI) lead to pathological 'remodelling' of the ventricle with dilatation and impaired contractility, one measure of which is a reduced ejection fraction (EF), that it is a sign of LV systolic dysfunction [10, 11].

What characterizes untreated systolic dysfunction is progressive worsening of these changes over time, with increasing enlargement of the LV and decline in EF. Two mechanisms that underlie these events: the occurrence of further events leading to additional myocyte death (e.g. recurrent MI) and the systemic responses induced by the decline in systolic function, particularly neurohumoral activation. Two key neurohumoral systems activated in HF are the renin–angiotensin–aldosterone system and sympathetic nervous system. Initially this neuro-hormonal mechanisms have a compensatory function, aimed at maintaining an adequate perfusion to vital organs, but in the long term influence a number of physiologic abnormalities counterproductive as the retention of sodium and water, peripheral vasoconstriction and degenerative processes of myocardial muscle. In addition to causing further myocardial injury, these systemic responses have detrimental effects on the blood vessels, kidneys, muscles, bone marrow, lungs, and liver, and create a pathophysiological "vicious cycle" (Fig. 2.6), accounting for many of the clinical features of the HF syndrome, including myocardial electrical instability. Interruption of these two key processes is the basis of much of the effective treatment of HF [10, 11].

In this contest it is clear that the renin-angiotensin system (RAS) plays a central role in the pathophysiology of HF. Therefore to know the mechanisms that underlie this system is an important element to understand and choose the best therapeutic strategy for HF.

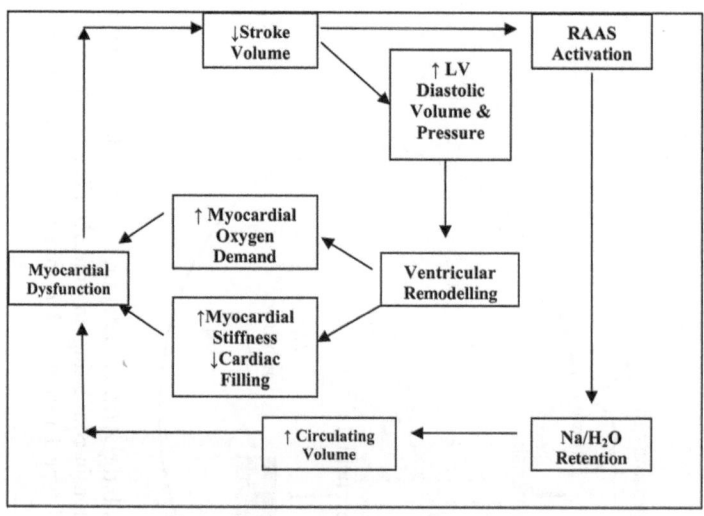

FIG. 2.6 The "vicious cycle" of the HF

The Renin-Angiotensin System

The RAS contributes in the contest of the HF to the increase of the peripheral vascular tone and hydrosaline retention concomitantly with the activation of the sympathetic nervous system. The reduction in cardiac output that characterizes HF causes an increase in plasma renin activity, levels of angiotensin II and aldosterone, which contribute to the development of the adverse effects that characterize HF. In Fig. 2.7 are depicted the different routes of production of angiotensin II which results from the activation of the system over that in circulating level also by an activation of the same at the tissue level, with local production of angiotensin II capable of performing a action vasoactive and trophic. The extent of activation of plasma ACE may reflect incompletely and partially the corresponding tissue activity in particular in patients with HF. Infact in this patient, from the very early stages, it could be observed a predominant local activation of the RAS with production of angiotensin II, even for alternative ways of

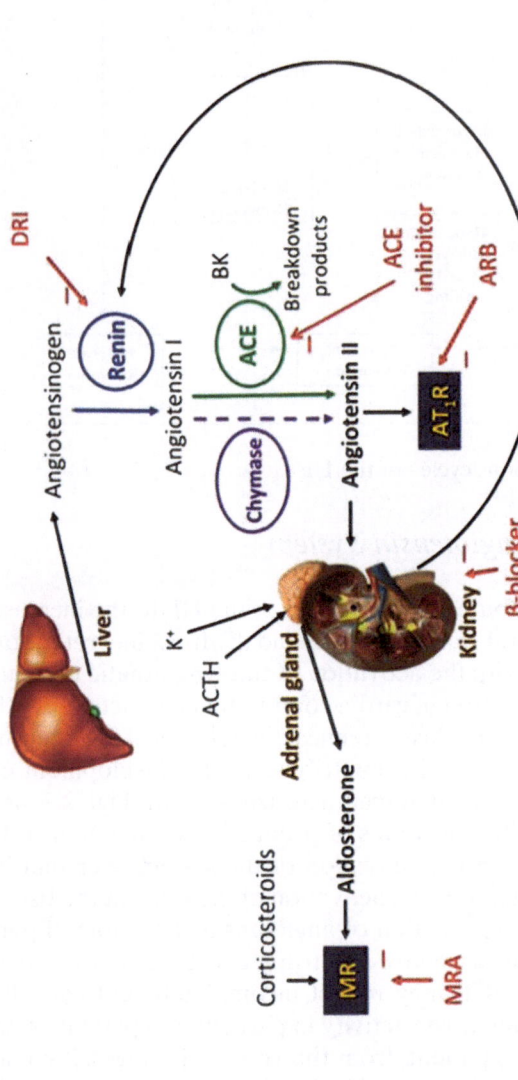

Fig. 2.7 The classical renin–angiotensin–system. *DRI* direct renin inhibitor, *ARB* angiotensin receptor blocker, *MRA* mineralocorticoid receptor antagonist, *K⁺* potassium ion, *ACE* angiotensin converting enzyme, *ACTH* adrenocortico-tropic hormone (corticotropin), *BK* bradykinin, AT_1R angiotensin II type 1 receptor, *MR* mineralcorticoid receptor (From McMurray [12])

production and non-employees from the ACE (es. chimasi) that seem particularly important at the tissue level where they could be responsible for the production of angiotensin II by up to 90 %. The RAS is, as can be imagined, also activated in the heart, where it has been hypothesized to contribute to ventricular remodeling phenomena described in the previous paragraph. Indeed angiotensin II is able to stimulate the growth of cardiomyocytes, in turn facilitated by the release of norepinephrine induced by angiotensin II at the level of the sympathetic nerve endings. The biological actions of angiotensin II are realized through the interaction with 4 subtypes of receptors called AT1-AT4, but at present most of the effects of angiotensin II appear mediated by the AT1 receptor, while for the AT2 receptor have been hypothesized anti-proliferative and vasodilators effects. The blockade of the AT1 receptor inhibits the action of angiotensin II at the receptor level, and allows a more efficient blockade of angiotensin II. In particular, one of the dominant effects of angiotensin II is represented by the stimulus to the production of aldosterone which has assumed great importance in patients with HF because of its ability to stimulate the reabsorption of sodium, but especially to induce the development of myocardial fibrosis with consequent the progression of myocardial structural alterations described in the previous paragraph. These changes are directly related to the progression of HF in hemodynamic level.

Focus on Blockade of the Renin–Angiotensin System

The objectives of the treatment of HF are varied and represented by the reduction of the symptoms, the prevention of the progression of the disease, by improving the quality of life, reduction in the frequency of hospitalization and especially by the prolongation of survival. In particular, the availability of drugs able to effectively interfere with the neurohumoral activation has allowed antagonize or modulate some of these systems to localization cardiac and extra-cardiac and responsible for the onset, the clinical expression and progression of the disease. In this context, ACE inhibitors represent the class of drugs most widely used among those used in the treatment of HF.

The clinical efficacy of ACE inhibitors follows to the unique mechanism of action that is articulated in an inhibition of the production of angiotensin II (potent vasoconstrictor and growth factor) which is associated with an inhibition of the degradation of the vasodilator bradykinin features of property resulting from the release of nitric oxide and prostacyclin. ACE inhibitors also reduce the activity of the sympathetic nervous system by inhibiting the action of angiotensin II which is capable of promoting the release of norepinephrine and inhibit the resorption (re-uptake). In addition, drugs of this class cause an increase in the density of the ß-adrenergic receptors (through mechanisms of up-regulation) and improve the heart rate variability, the response of the baroreceptor and autonomic function (including the vagal tone).

ACE inhibitors also exhibit antiproliferative effects (reduction of vascular and cardiac hypertrophy and extracellular matrix proliferation) and reduce ventricular remodelling after myocardial infarction [13, 14]. In the hypertrophied heart reduce cardiac hypertrophy and improve diastolic function.

Moreover ACE inhibitors decrease renal vascular resistances and increase renal blood flow and promote Na^+ and water excretion by the relatively greater effect in dilating postglomerular efferent than afferent arterioles, leading to a reduction in glomerular capillary hydrostatic pressure and glomerular filtration rate (GFR) [15]. So prevent progression of microalbuminuria to overt proteinuria [16], attenuate the progression of renal insufficiency in patients with a variety of non-diabetic nephropathies [17] and prevent or delay the progression of nephropathy in patients with insulindependent diabetes mellitus [18, 19].

In most patients ACE inhibitors are well tolerated, however, several adverse reactions may occur. They can also appear at any time during treatment, even in patients already chronically treated with ACE inhibitors. The most common adverse reaction associated with their use in the elderly population is orthostatic hypotension (prevalence, ~ 50 %), especially during the first few days of treatment or after a dose increase. Dry cough appears in 5–10 % of patients, this is the most common adverse reaction associated with increased concentration of kinins, and is not dose-dependent. If the cough persists and interferes with quality of life, therapy with ACE inhibitors may be suspended and replaced by the administration of angiotensin II receptor blockers. Hyperkalemia due to a decrease in aldosterone secretion is rarely found in patients with normal renal function but it is relatively common in those with congestive HF and in the elderly. This side effect is also more frequent in patients with renal impairment, diabetes, receiving either K^+ or potassium K^+-sparing diuretics, heparin or Non-Steroidal Anti-Inflammatory Drugs (NSAIDs). Angioedema is a rare but potentially life-threatening and appears related to an accumulation of bradykinin. Symptoms range from mild gastrointestinal disturbances to severe dyspnea and death. Finally ACE inhibitors, taken during the second or third trimester of pregnancy, may present some teratogenic effects.

Trials That Support the Use of Angiotensing-Converting Enzyme Inhibitors

The evidence supporting the use of ACE inhibitors in patients with HF is based on the results of wide prospective clinical studies (Fig. 2.8). This trials have demonstrated and repeatedly confirmed that ACE inhibitors are effective in reducing morbidity and mortality and are also able to improve the quality of life in patients with asymptomatic LV dysfunction or suffering from a overt congestive HF resulting from a reduced systolic function of the LV or when it is a result of a MI.

Trial	Year	N.pz	Class NYHA	Follow up (months)	Admission (RR, %)	Total deaths (RR, %)
CONSENSUS (enalapril 18.4 mg/die)	1987	253	IV	6	NA	↓ 27 p=.003
SOLVD-T (enalapril 16.6 mg/die)	1991	2569	II-III	41	↓ 26 p<.0001	↓ 16 p=.0036
SOLVD-P (enalapril 16.7 mg/die)	1992	428	I-III	37	↓ 44 p<.001	↓ 8 p=NA
SAVE (captopril18-150 mg/die)	1992	2231	I	42	↓ 22 p=.019	↓ 19 p=.019
AIRE (ramipril 15-10 mg/die)	1993	2006	II-III	15	NA	↓ 27 p=.002
TRACE (trandolapril 1-4 mg/die)	1995	1749	I-IV	24	NA	↓ 22 p=.001
SMILE (zofenopril 15-60 mg/die)	1995	1556	I-IV	12	NA	↓ 29 p=.011

FIG. 2.8 Main trials on ACE inhibitors. *NA* not available

Two key randomized controlled trials [Cooperative North Scandinavian Enalapril Survival Study (CONSENSUS) [20] and Studies of Left Ventricular Dysfunction (SOLVD)-Treatment] [21] assigned about 2,800 patients with mild to severely symptomatic HF to placebo or enalapril. This trials show how the addition of enalapril to conventional therapy in patients with severe congestive HF can reduce mortality and improve symptoms. The beneficial effect on mortality is due to a reduction in death from the progression of HF (Fig. 2.9).

In particular the CONSENSUS evaluate the influence of the angiotensin-converting-enzyme inhibitor enalapril (2.5–40 mg per day) on the prognosis of severe congestive HF (New York Heart Association [NYHA] functional class IV). The trial randomizes 253 patients in a double-blind study to receive either placebo (n = 126) or enalapril (n = 127). Conventional treatment for HF, including the use of other vasodilators, was continued in both groups. Follow-up averaged 188 days (range, 1 day to 20 months). The crude mortality at the end of 6 months (primary end point) was 26 % in the enalapril group and 44 % in the placebo group: a reduction of 40 % (P = 0.002). Mortality was reduced by 31 % at 1 year (P = 0.001). By the end of the study, there had been 68 deaths in the placebo group and 50 in the enalapril group: a

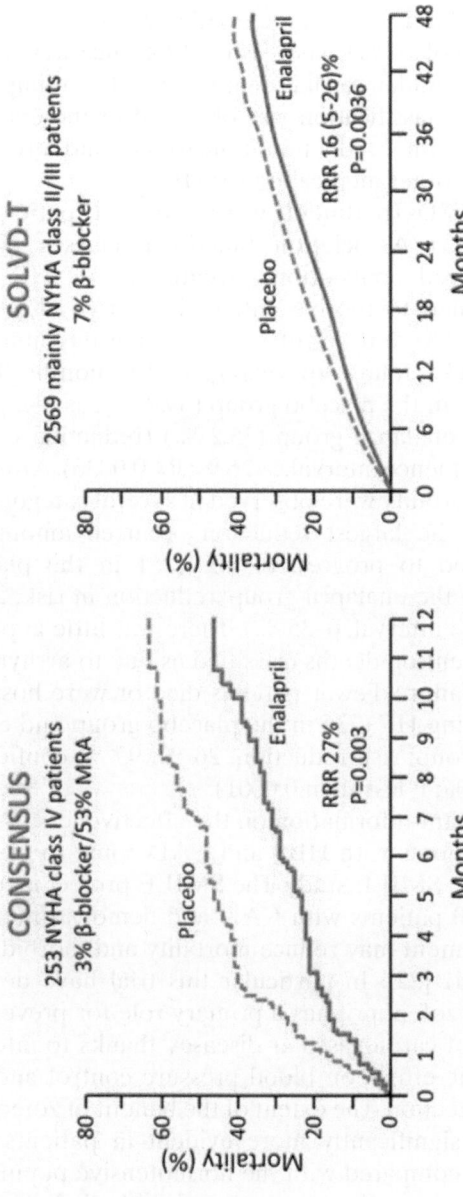

FIG. 2.9 Trials comparing an angiotensin-converting enzyme (ACE) inhibitor to placebo in patients with systolic heart failure. Outcome is cumulative mortality (From The CONSENSUS Trial Study Group [20] and The SOLVD Investigators [21])

reduction of 27 % (P = 0.003). The entire reduction in total mortality was found to be among patients with progressive HF (a reduction of 50 %), whereas no difference was seen in the incidence of sudden cardiac death. A significant improvement in NYHA classification was observed in the enalapril group, together with a reduction in heart size and a reduced requirement for other medication for HF.

In the SOLVD-Treatment were enrolled patients in New York Heart Association functional classes II and III. They received conventional treatment for HF were randomly assigned to receive either placebo (n = 1,284) or enalapril (n = 1,285) at doses of 2.5–20 mg per day in a double-bind trial. The follow-up averaged 41.4 months. There were 510 deaths in the placebo group (39.7 %), as compared with 452 in the enalapril group (35.2 %) (reduction in risk, 16 %; 95 % confidence interval, 5–26 %; P = 0.0036). Although reductions in mortality were observed in several categories of cardiac deaths, the largest reduction occurred among the deaths attributed to progressive HF (251 in the placebo group vs. 209 in the enalapril group; reduction in risk, 22 %; 95 % confidence interval, 6–35 %). There was little apparent effect of treatment on deaths classified as due to arrhythmia without pump failure. Fewer patients died or were hospitalized for worsening HF (736 in the placebo group and 613 in the enalapril group; risk reduction, 26 %; 95 % confidence interval, 18–34 %; P less than 0.0001).

Other important information on the effectiveness of ACE inhibitors in patients with HBP and CAD come to us from the results of the SMILE study. The SMILE project involved more than 3,500 patients with CAD and demonstrated that zofenopril treatment may reduce mortality and morbidity in patients with MI [22]. In particular this trial have demonstrated that the zofenopril has a primary role for prevention and treatment of cardiovascular diseases, thanks to interesting anti-ischemic effect, on blood pressure control and cardiovascular protection. The extent of the benefit of zofenopril treatment was significantly more evident in patients with history of HBP compared with the normotensive population (Fig. 2.10) [23] as well as in patients with diabetes [24]

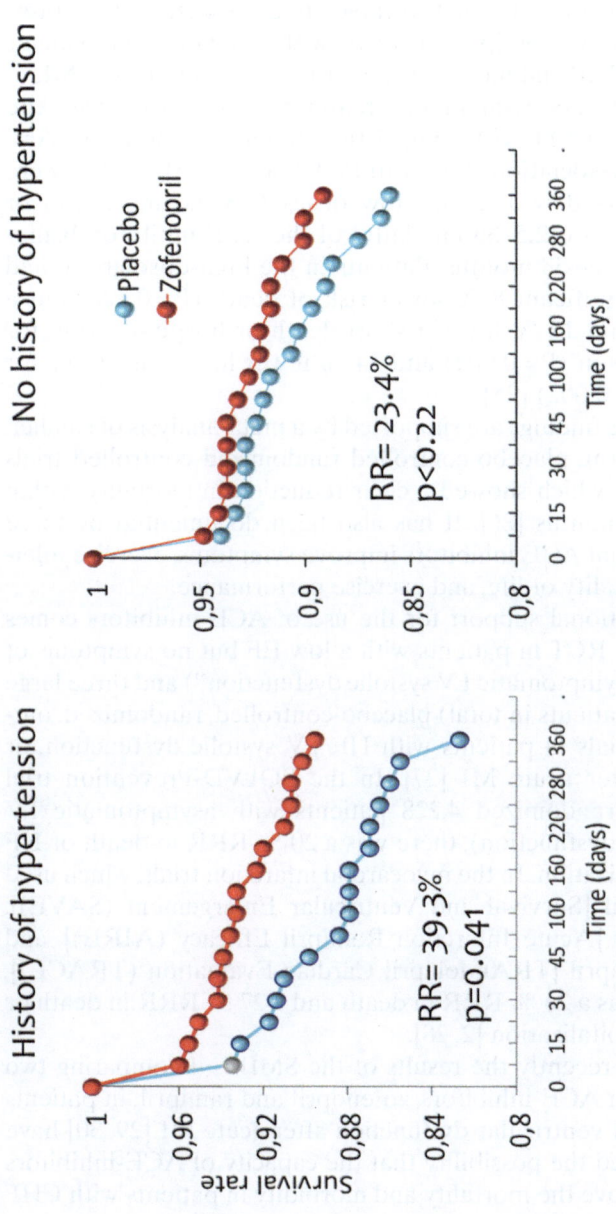

Fig. 2.10 Role of Zofenopril in reducing the incidence of events by approximately 40% in subjects with a history of hypertension (From SMILE Study Investigators [23])

probably owing to the favorable effects of better blood pressure and glycol-lipidic control with zofenopril in patients where HBP and metabolic abnormalities complicated MI.

In the Assessment of Treatment with Lisinopril And Survival (ATLAS) trial, 3,164 patients with New York Heart Association class II to IV HF and an EF ≤ 30 % were randomized with either low doses (2.5–5.0 mg daily) or high doses (32.5–35 mg daily) of the ACE inhibitor, lisinopril, for 39–58 months. Patients in the high-dose group had a nonsignificant 8 % lower risk of death (P = 0.128) but a significant 12 % lower risk of death or hospitalization for any reason (P = 0.002) and 24 % fewer hospitalizations for HF (P = 0.002) [25].

These findings are supported by a meta-analysis of smaller, short-term, placebo-controlled randomized controlled trials (RCTs), which showed a clear reduction in mortality within only 3 months [26]. It has also been documented by these RCTs that ACE inhibitors improve symptoms, exercise tolerance, quality of life, and exercise performance.

Additional support for the use of ACE inhibitors comes from an RCT in patients with a low EF but no symptoms of HF ("asymptomatic LV systolic dysfunction") and three large (5,966 patients in total) placebo-controlled, randomized, outcome trials in patients with HF, LV systolic dysfunction, or both after acute MI [27]. In the SOLVD-Prevention trial (which randomized 4,228 patients with asymptomatic LV systolic dysfunction), there was a 20 % RRR in death or HF hospitalization. In the myocardial infarction trials, which used captopril [Survival and Ventricular Enlargement (SAVE)], ramipril [Acute Infarction Ramipril Efficacy (AIRE)], and trandolapril [TRAndolapril Cardiac Evaluation (TRACE)], there was a 26 % RRR in death and a 27 % RRR in death or HF hospitalization [2, 28].

Very recently the results of the SMILE 4 comparing two different ACE-inhibitors, zofenopril and ramipril, in patients with left ventricular dysfunction after acute MI [29, 30] have suggested the possibility that the capacity of ACE-inhibitors to improve the mortality and morbidity in patients with CHF can be significantly affected by the structural properties of the ACE-inhibitors. In particular the cumulative incidence of death and hospitalization for CV causes has resulted significantly reduced in patients treated with zofenopril whose anti-ischemic properties along with a more effective tissue penetration and antioxidant effect may have some remarkable impact on the protection of cardiac structure and function. The observations of the SMILE 4 study have been confirmed in a population of elderly patients with chronic CHF [19] where again the treatment with zofenopril was associated with a better survival in comparison to ramipril after adjustment for the most important confounding factors. These data open a new perspective in the treatment of patients with CHF where the choice of the ACE-inhibitor should not exclusively based on the main mechanism of action but also on the possibility that some additive properties can play some role by improving the capacity of the drugs to reach the tissue targets and by exerting some additional cardioprotective effects that can improve left ventricular function beyond the average expected by the pharmacological class.

ACE-Inhibitors Compared with Angiotensin Receptor Blockers

The clinical efficacy of ACE inhibitors has been compared with that of direct angiotensin-II receptor antagonists in several trials.

The second losartan in HF survival study (ELITE-2) showed equivalent effect on mortality and morbidity between losartan and captopril and less adverse events in losartan: mortality in 3,152 patients with chronic HF was similar in losartan and captopril, after a follow-up of 555 days (11.7 % vs. 10.4 %, respectively) [31].

In the Optimal Trial in Myocardial Infarction with the Angiotensin II Antagonist Losartan (OPTIMAAL) 5,477 patients, with confirmed acute MI and HF during the acute phase or a new Q-wave anterior infarction or reinfarction, were randomly to receive losartan or captopril. The trial show how there isn't a non-significant difference in total mortality in favour of captopril (18 % and 16 % respectively) [32].

In the VALIANT trial 15,703 patients with MI complicated by LV systolic dysfunction, HF or both were randomised to receive captopril or valsartan or the combination of both drugs. The trial shows how valsartan is as effective as captopril between the three groups with regard to mortality or other clinical outcomes [33].

On the contrary, in the Candesartan in HF: Assessment of Reduction in Mortality and morbidity (CHARM)-added trial, the addition of candesartan to an ACE inhibitors lead to a clinical important reduction in relevant cardiovascular events in patients with CHF and reduced left-ventricular ejection fraction, although mortality was not reduced [34]. Since no differences have been demonstrated to date between ACE inhibitors and angiotensin-II blockers, ACE inhibitors should remain the first-choice treatment in patients with HF [35].

Use of the ACE Inhibitors in the Hearth Failure: ESC and ACCF/AHA Guidelines

According to the **ESC (European Society of Cardiology) guidelines for the diagnosis and treatment of acute and chronic HF**, an ACE inhibitor is recommended, in addition to a beta-blocker, for all patients with an EF ≤40 % to reduce the risk of HF hospitalization and the risk of premature death (class of recommendation I, level of evidence A) [2, 20, 21, 34–36].

From the ESC guidelines [35]:

- indication for a patients should get an ACE inhibitor: EF ≤40 %, irrespective of symptoms;
- contraindications: a history of angioedema, bilateral renal artery stenosis, serum potassium concentration >5.0 mmol/L, serum creatinine >220 mmol/L (~2.5 mg/dL), severe aortic stenosis.

	Starting dose (mg)	Target dose (mg)
ACE inhibitor		
Captopril[a]	6.25 t.i.d.	50 t.i.d.
Enalapril	2.5 b.i.d.	10–20 b.i.d.
Lisinopril[b]	2.5–5.0 o.d.	20–35 o.d.
Ramipril	2.5 o.d.	5 b.i.d.
Trandolapril[a]	0.5 o.d.	4 o.d.

FIG. 2.11 Evidence-based doses of disease-modifying drugs used in key randomized trials. [a]Indicates an ACE inhibitor where the dosing target is derived from post-myocardial infarction trials. [b]Indicates drugs where a higher dose has been shown to reduce morbidity–mortality compared with a lower dose of the same drug, but there is no substantive placebo-controlled randomized controlled trial and the optimum dose is uncertain. *b.i.d.* bis in die (twice daily), *o.d.* omni die (once every day), *t.i.d.* ter in die (three times daily)

- First to use an ACE inhibitor in HF is important to check renal function and serum electrolytes. Within 1–2 weeks of starting treatment can be useful re-check renal function and serum electrolytes.
- Dose up-titration (Fig. 2.11):
  - Consider dose up-titration after 2–4 weeks. Do not increase dose if significant worsening of renal function or hyperkalaemia. Re-check renal function and serum electrolytes 1 and 4 weeks after increasing dose. More rapid dose up-titration can be carried out in patients in hospital or otherwise closely supervised, tolerability permitting.
  - In the absence of above problems, aim for evidence-based target dose or maximum tolerated dose.
  - Re-check renal function and serum electrolytes in the following months.
- Potential adverse effects:
  - Worsening renal function: if necessary, reduce ACE inhibitor dose or discontinue.

- Hyperkalaemia: control if the patient takes other agents causing hyperkalaemia, e.g. potassium supplements and potassium-sparing diuretics, e.g. amiloride, and stop.
- Symptomatic hypotension (e.g. dizziness) is common, often improves with time, and patients should be reassured. Consider reducing the dose of diuretics and other hypotensive agents. Asymptomatic hypotension does not require intervention.
- Cough: if an ACE inhibitor causes a troublesome cough, switch to an angiotensin receptor blockers (ARB).

In the combination therapy must pay attention to some associations, infact some treatments may cause harm in patients with symptomatic (NYHA class II-IV) systolic HF: the addition of an ARB or renin inhibitor, to the combination of an ACE inhibitor AND a MRA is NOT recommended because of the risk of renal dysfunction and hyperkalaemia. (Class III, Level C).

In acute HF after stabilization of the clinical, in patients with an EF ≤40 % an ACE inhibitor is recommended to reduce the risk of death, recurrent MI, and hospitalization for HF. (Class I, Level A).

Management of other particular conditions and co-morbidity in HF with preserved EF:

- In patients with ventricular arrhythmias it is recommended that treatment with an ACE inhibitor (or ARB), beta-blocker, and MRA should be optimized. (Class I, Level A).
- Dysglycemia and diabetes are very common in HF, and diabetes is associated with poorer functional status and worse prognosis. So in this patients, diabetes may be prevented by treatment with ACE inhibitors [36].
- For the treatment of HBP in patients with symptomatic HF (NYHA functional class II–IV) and LV systolic dysfunction one or more of an ACE inhibitor (or ARB), beta-blocker, and MRA is recommended as first, second, and third-line therapy, respectively, because of their associated

benefits (reducing the risk of HF hospitalization and reducing the risk of premature death). (Class I, Level A)
- In patient with kidney dysfunction and cardiorenal syndrome the GFR is reduced in most patients with HF, especially if advanced, and renal function is a powerful independent predictor of prognosis in HF. So the ACE inhibitors frequently can cause a fall in GFR, although any reduction is usually small and should not lead to treatment discontinuation unless marked.

On the other side of the ocean also the **ACCF/AHA (American College of Cardiology Foundation/American Heart Association) guidelines of the HF** recognize an important role of ACE inhibitors [37].

In this guidelines patients are classified according to four stages, which reflects the growing appreciation for the importance of the prevention of HF:

- Stage A: patients at high risk for developing HF but without structural heart disease or symptoms of HF;
- Stage B: patients with structural heart disease but without signs or symptoms of HF;
- Stage C: patients with structural heart disease with prior or current symptoms of HF;
- Stage D: patients with end-stage disease who require specialized treatment strategies (refractory HF).

In the *Stage A* ACE inhibitors are recommended for the treatment of elevated blood pressure, diabetes mellitus, obesity, dyslipidemia and vascular risk.

In the *Stage B* in all patients with a recent or remote history of MI or acute coronary syndrome and reduced EF, ACE inhibitors should be used to prevent symptomatic HF and reduce mortality. (Class I, Level A). And they should be used in all patients with a reduced EF to prevent symptomatic HF, even if they do not have a history of MI. (Class I, Level A).

Current evidence supports the use of ACE inhibitors and (to a lower level of evidence) beta-blocker therapy to impede maladaptive LV remodeling in patients with stage B HF and low LVEF to improve mortality and morbidity [38]. At 3-year follow-up, those patients treated with ACE inhibitors demonstrated combined endpoints of reduced hospitalization or death, a benefit that extended up to a 12-year follow-up [39].

ACE inhibitors are also recommended in patients with HF with reduced EF (HFrEF) and current or prior symptoms (*Stage C*), unless contraindicated, to reduce morbidity and mortality. (Class I, Level A).

Their use in patients with HBP is also reasonable to control blood pressure in patients with HF preserved EF (HFpEF). (Class IIa, Level C)

ACE inhibitors can reduce the risk of death and reduce hospitalization in HFrEF.

- Patients should not be given an ACE inhibitor if they have experienced life threatening adverse reactions (i.e., angioedema) during previous medication exposure or if they are pregnant or plan to become pregnant.
- Dose up-titration:
  - clinicians should prescribe an ACE inhibitor with caution if the patient has very low systemic blood pressures (systolic blood pressure <80 mmHg), markedly increased serum levels of creatinine (>3 mg/dL), bilateral renal artery stenosis, or elevated levels of serum potassium (>5.0 mEq/L).
  - Treatment with an ACE inhibitor should be initiated at low doses, followed by gradual dose increments if lower doses have been well tolerated.
  - Renal function and serum potassium should be assessed within 1–2 weeks of initiation of therapy and periodically thereafter.

- The majority of the adverse reactions of ACE inhibitors can be attributed to the two principal pharmacological actions of these drugs: angiotensin suppression and kinin potentiation. Other types of adverse effects may also occur (e.g., rash, taste disturbances, cough). With the use of ACE inhibitors, particular care should be given to the patient's volume status, renal function, and concomitant medications.

In controlled clinical trials that were designed to evaluate survival, the dose of the ACE inhibitor was not determined by a patient's therapeutic response but was increased until the predetermined target dose was reached [20, 21, 24]. Clinicians should attempt to use doses that have been shown to reduce the risk of cardiovascular events in clinical trials. If these target doses of an ACE inhibitor cannot be used or are poorly tolerated, intermediate doses should be used with the expectation that there are likely to be only small differences in efficacy between low and high doses. Abrupt withdrawal of treatment with an ACE inhibitor can lead to clinical deterioration and should be avoided.

In conclusion, ACE-inhibitors are a cornerstone in the treatment of congestive heart failure and their favorable impact affect both mortality and rate of hospital admission thereby improving the overall prognosis and the economic budget. The advantage of ACE-inhibitors is related to their activity of blockade of the over-activated neuro-humoral system both in the plasma and at the tissue level. In addition the more integrated mechanism of action of

References

1. Dickstein K, Cohen-Solal A, Filippatos G, McMurray JJ, Ponikowski P, Poole-Wilson PA, Stromberg A, van Veldhuisen DJ, Atar D, Hoes AW, Keren A, Mebazaa A, Nieminen M, Priori SG, Swedberg K. ESC guidelines for the diagnosis and treatment of acute and chronic heart failure 2008: the Task Force for the diagnosis and treatment of acute and chronic heart failure 2008 of the European Society of Cardiology. Developed in collaboration with the Heart Failure Association of the ESC (HFA) and endorsed by the European Society of Intensive Care Medicine (ESICM). Eur J Heart Fail. 2008;10:933–89.
2. Guidelines ESC. for the diagnosis and treatment of acute and chronic heart failure 2012: The Task Force for the Diagnosis and Treatment of Acute and Chronic Heart Failure 2012 of the European Society of Cardiology. Developed in collaboration with the Heart Failure Association (HFA) of the ESC. Eur Heart J. 2012;33(14):1787–847.

3. Mosterd A, Hoes AW. Clinical epidemiology of heart failure. Heart. 2007;93:1137–46.

4. Cleland JG, Swedberg K, Follath F, Komajda M, Cohen-Solal A, Aguilar JC, Dietz R, Gavazzi A, Hobbs R, Korewicki J, Madeira HC, Moiseyev VS, Preda I, van Gilst WH, Widimsky J, Freemantle N, Eastaugh J, Mason J. Study Group on Diagnosis of the Working Group on Heart Failure of the European Society of Cardiology. The EuroHeart Failure survey programme – a survey on the quality of care among patients with heart failure in Europe. Part 1: patient characteristics and diagnosis. Eur Heart J. 2003;24(5):442–63.

5. Stewart S, MacIntyre K, Hole DJ, Capewell S, McMurray JJ. More 'malignant' than cancer? Five-year survival following a first admission for heart failure. Eur J Heart Fail. 2001;3:315–22.

6. Stewart S, Ekman I, Ekman T, Oden A, Rosengren A. Population impact of heart failure and the most common forms of cancer: a study of 1 162 309 hospital cases in Sweden (1988 to 2004). Circ Cardiovasc Qual Outcomes. 2010;3:573–80.

7. Jhund PS, Macintyre K, Simpson CR, Lewsey JD, Stewart S, Redpath A, Chalmers JW, Capewell S, McMurray JJ. Long-term trends in first hospitalization for heart failure and subsequent survival between 1986 and 2003: a population study of 5.1 million people. Circulation. 2009;119:515–23.

8. Ackerman MJ, Priori SG, Willems S, Berul C, Brugada R, Calkins H, Camm AJ, Ellinor PT, Gollob M, Hamilton R, Hershberger RE, Judge DP, Le Marec H, McKenna WJ, Schulze-Bahr E, Semsarian C, Towbin JA, Watkins H, Wilde A, Wolpert C, Zipes DP. HRS/EHRA expert consensus statement on the state of genetic testing for the channelopathies and cardiomyopathies: this document was developed as a partnership between the Heart Rhythm Society (HRS) and the European Heart Rhythm Association (EHRA). Heart Rhythm. 2011;8:1308–39.

9. Survey on heart failure in Italian hospital cardiology units. Results of the SEOSI study. SEOSI Investigators. Eur Heart J. 1997;18(9):1457–64.

10. McMurray JJ. Clinical practice. Systolic heart failure. N Engl J Med. 2010;362:228–38.

11. Shah AM, Mann DL. In search of new therapeutic targets and strategies for heart failure: recent advances in basic science. Lancet. 2011;378:704–12.

12. McMurray JJ. CONSENSUS to EMPHASIS: the overwhelming evidence which makes blockade of the renin-angiotensin-

aldosterone system the cornerstone of therapy for systolic heart failure. Eur J Heart Fail. 2011;13(9):929–36.

13. Paul M, Ganten D. The molecular basis of cardiovascular hypertrophy: the role of the renin–angiotensin system. J Cardiovasc Pharmacol. 1992;19 Suppl 5:S51–8.

14. Schiffrin E, Deng L. Comparison of effects of angiotensin I-converting enzyme inhibition and b-blockade for 2 years on function of small arteries from hypertensive patients. Hypertension. 1995;25:699–703.

15. Matsuda H, Hayashi K, Arakawa K. Zonal heterogeneity in action of angiotensin-converting enzyme inhibitor on renal microcirculation: role of intrarenal bradykinin. J Am Soc Nephrol. 1999;10:2272–82.

16. Keane WF, Shapiro BE. Renal protective effects of angiotensin-converting enzyme inhibition. Am J Cardiol. 1990;65:49I–53.

17. Ruggenenti P, Perna A, Gherardi G, et al. Renoprotective properties of ACE-inhibition in non-diabetic nephropathies and non-nephrotic proteinuria. Lancet. 1999;354:359–64.

18. Lewis EJ, Hunsicker LG, Bain RP, et al. The effect of angiotensinconverting enzyme inhibition on diabetic nephropathy. N Engl J Med. 1993;329:1456–62.

19. Pitt B, Poole-Wilson PA, Segl R, on behalf of the ELITE II Investigators. Effect of losartan compared with captopril on mortality in patients with symptomatic heart failure: randomised trial – the Losartan Heart Failure Survival Study ELITE II. Lancet. 2000;355:1582–7.

20. Effects of enalapril on mortality in severe congestive heart failure. Results of the Cooperative North Scandinavian Enalapril Survival Study (CONSENSUS). The CONSENSUS Trial Study Group. N Engl J Med. 1987;316:1429–35.

21. Effect of enalapril on survival in patients with reduced left ventricular ejection fractions and congestive heart failure. The SOLVD Investigators. N Engl J Med. 1991;325:293–302.

22. Ambrosioni E, Borghi C, Magnani B. The effect of the angiotensin-converting-enzyme inhibitor zofenopril on mortality and morbidity after anterior myocardial infarction. The Survival of Myocardial Infarction Long-Term Evaluation (SMILE) Study Investigators. N Engl J Med. 1995;332:80–5.

23. Borghi C, Bacchelli S, Esposti DD, Bignamini A, Magnani B, Ambrosioni E. Effects of the administration of an angiotensin-converting enzyme inhibitor during the acute phase of myocardial infarction in patients with arterial hypertension. SMILE

Study Investigators. Survival of Myocardial Infarction Long-term Evaluation. Am J Hypertens. 1999;12(7):665–72.

24. Borghi C, Bacchelli S, Esposti DD, Ambrosioni E, SMILE Study. Effects of the early ACE inhibition in diabetic nonthrombolyzed patients with anterior acute myocardial infarction. Diabetes Care. 2003;26:1862–8.

25. Packer M, Poole-Wilson PA, Armstrong PW, Cleland JG, Horowitz JD, Massie BM, Ryden L, Thygesen K, Uretsky BF. Comparative effects of low and high doses of the angiotensin-converting enzyme inhibitor, lisinopril, on morbidity and mortality in chronic heart failure. ATLAS Study Group. Circulation. 1999;100:2312–8.

26. Garg R, Yusuf S. Overview of randomized trials of angiotensin-converting enzyme inhibitors on mortality and morbidity in patients with heart failure. Collaborative Group on ACE Inhibitor Trials. JAMA. 1995;273:1450–6.

27. The SOLVD Investigators. Effect of enalapril on mortality and the development of heart failure in asymptomatic patients with reduced left ventricular ejection fractions. N Engl J Med. 1992;327:685–91.

28. Flather MD, Yusuf S, Kober L, Pfeffer M, Hall A, Murray G, Torp-Pedersen C, Ball S, Pogue J, Moye L, Braunwald E. Long-term ACE-inhibitor therapy in patients with heart failure or left-ventricular dysfunction: a systematic overview of data from individual patients. ACE-Inhibitor Myocardial Infarction Collaborative Group. Lancet. 2000;355:1575–81.

29. Borghi C, Ambrosioni E, Novo S, Vinereanu D, Ambrosio G, SMILE-4 Working Party. Comparison between zofenopril and ramipril in combination with acetylsalicylic acid in patients with left ventricular systolic dysfunction after acute myocardial infarction: results of a randomized, double-blind, parallel-group, multicenter, European study (SMILE-4). Clin Cardiol. 2012;35:416–23.

30. Borghi C, Cosentino ER, Rinaldi ER, Cicero AF. Effect of zofenopril and ramipril on cardiovascular mortality in patients with chronic heart failure. Am J Cardiol. 2013;112(1): 90–93.

31. Dickstein K, Kjekshus J, OPTIMAAL Steering Committee for the OPTIMAAL Study Group. Effects of losartan and captopril on mortality and morbidity high-risk patients after acute myocardial infarction: the OPTIMAAL randomised trial. Lancet. 2002;360:752–60.

32. Pfeffer MA, McMurray JJV, Velasquez EJ, et al., for the Valsartan in Acute Myocardial Infarction Trial Investigators. Valsartan, captopril, or both in myocardial infarction complicated by heart failure, left ventricular dysfunction, or both. N Engl J Med. 2003;349:1893–906.

33. McMurray JJV, Ostergren J, Swedberg K, et al. Effects of candesartan in patients with chronic heart failure and reduced left-ventricular systolic function taking angiotensin converting-enzyme inhibitors: the CHARM-Added trial. Lancet. 2003;362:767–71.

34. López-Sendón J, Swedberg K, McMurray J, Tamargo J, Maggioni AP, Dargie H, Tendera M, Waagstein F, Kjekshus J, Lechat P, Torp-Pedersen C, Task Force on ACE-inhibitors of the European Society of Cardiology. Expert consensus document on angiotensin converting enzyme inhibitors in cardiovascular disease. The Task Force on ACE-inhibitors of the European Society of Cardiology. Eur Heart J. 2004;25(16):1454–70.

35. Guidelines ESC. for the diagnosis and treatment of acute and chronic heart failure 2008: the Task Force for the Diagnosis and Treatment of Acute and Chronic Heart Failure 2008 of the European Society of Cardiology. Developed in collaboration with the Heart Failure Association of the ESC (HFA) and endorsed by the European Society of Intensive Care Medicine (ESICM). Eur Heart J. 2008;29(19):2388–442.

36. McMurray JJ, Holman RR, Haffner SM, Bethel MA, Holzhauer B, Hua TA, Belenkov Y, Boolell M, Buse JB, Buckley BM, Chacra AR, Chiang FT, Charbonnel B, Chow CC, Davies MJ, Deedwania P, Diem P, Einhorn D, Fonseca V, Fulcher GR, Gaciong Z, Gaztambide S, Giles T, Horton E, Ilkova H, Jenssen T, Kahn SE, Krum H, Laakso M, Leiter LA, Levitt NS, Mareev V, Martinez F, Masson C, Mazzone T, Meaney E, Nesto R, Pan C, Prager R, Raptis SA, Rutten GE, Sandstroem H, Schaper F, Scheen A, Schmitz O, Sinay I, Soska V, Stender S, Tamas G, Tognoni G, Tuomilehto J, Villamil AS, Vozar J, Califf RM. Effect of valsartan on the incidence of diabetes and cardiovascular events. N Engl J Med. 2010;362:1477–90.

37. Yancy CW, Jessup M, Bozkurt B, Butler J, Casey Jr DE, Drazner MH, Fonarow GC, Geraci SA, Horwich T, Januzzi JL, Johnson MR, Kasper EK, Levy WC, Masoudi FA, McBride PE, McMurray JJ, Mitchell JE, Peterson PN, Riegel B, Sam F, Stevenson LW, Tang WH, Tsai EJ, Wilkoff BL. 2013 ACCF/AHA guideline for the management of heart failure: a report of the American

College of Cardiology Foundation/American Heart Association Task Force on Practice Guidelines. J Am Coll Cardiol. 2013;62(16):e147–239.

38. Colucci WS, Elkayam U, Horton DP, Abraham WT, Bourge RC, Johnson AD, Wagoner LE, Givertz MM, Liang CS, Neibaur M, Haught WH, LeJemtel TH. Intravenous nesiritide, a natriuretic peptide, in the treatment of decompensated congestive heart failure. Nesiritide Study Group. N Engl J Med. 2000;343(4):246–53.

39. Vasan RS, Beiser A, Seshadri S, et al. Residual lifetime risk for developing hypertension in middle-aged women and men: The Framingham Heart Study. JAMA. 2002;287:1003–10.

Chapter 3
Impact of Chronic Kidney Disease and Diabetes Mellitus on Choice of Renin Angiotensin System-Inhibitors in Patients with Hypertension and Heart Failure

Pantelis A. Sarafidis, Panagiotis I. Georgianos, Pantelis E. Zebekakis, and Athanasios J. Manolis

Introduction

Heart failure (HF) represents a complex clinical syndrome arising from any structural and functional cardiovascular alteration that affects ventricular filling or blood ejection [1]. Current epidemiological estimates on the burden of HF in the

P.A. Sarafidis, M.D., M.Sc., Ph.D.
Department of Nephrology, "Hippokration" General Hospital,
Aristotle University of Thessaloniki, Thessaloniki, Greece

P.I. Georgianos, M.D. • P.E. Zebekakis, M.D., Ph.D.
Section of Nephrology and Hypertension, 1st Department of Medicine,
Aristotle University of Thessaloniki, AHEPA University Hospital,
Thessaloniki, Greece

A.J. Manolis, M.D., Ph.D. (✉)
Department of Cardiology, Asklepeion General Hospital,
1 Vas. Pavlou Ave, Voula, Athens 16673, Greece
e-mail: ajmanol@otenet.gr

© Springer International Publishing Switzerland 2015   73
P. Perrone Filardi (ed.), *ACEi and ARBS in Hypertension
and Heart Failure*, Current Cardiovascular Therapy 5,
DOI 10.1007/978-3-319-09788-6_3

adult population of United States of America (USA) suggest that above 650,000 new cases of HF are diagnosed annually and that approximately 5.1 million adults in USA have clinically overt HF [2]. Prevalence rates of HF exhibited an increasing trend during the previous two decades and are anticipated to significantly worsen in the up-coming future [3, 4]. Importantly, development, persistence and progression of HF are well-documented risk factors of cardiovascular and all-cause mortality and despite the important progress in treatment, the absolute mortality rates for HF reach approximately 50 % within the first 5 years following the diagnosis [5, 6].

Hypertension is the most common chronic disorder worldwide and represents a well-established risk factor for the development of HF [7]. Large-scaled outcome trials in hypertension have provided a strong body of evidence that blood pressure (BP)-lowering is associated with an about 50 % reduction in the risk of incident HF and with beneficial impact on survival of HF patients [7]. On this basis, the American College of Cardiology Foundation/American Heart Association (ACCF/AHA) 2013 Guidelines [1] for the management of HF recommend adequate control of both systolic and diastolic BP as a major treatment effort towards cardiovascular risk reduction in these individuals. Antihypertensive drugs proven to be effective and recommended by current international guidelines as first-line treatment in patients with hypertension and HF include angiotensin converting enzyme-inhibitors (ACEI), angiotensin receptor blockers (ARBs), β-blockers and diuretic agents [1]. However, large proportions of HF patients suffer concomitantly from other co-morbid conditions, such as chronic kidney disease (CKD) and diabetes mellitus (DM), which can substantially influence the choice of the appropriate BP-lowering regimen.

Selection of antihypertensive treatment has to take into account the effects of different antihypertensive drug classes on metabolic and other related parameters as well as the specific indications and contra-indications of BP-lowering drugs and combinations depending on patients' co-morbid conditions. Thus, in patients with diabetic or non-diabetic proteinuric

CKD, ACEI and ARBs are currently recommended as antihypertensive agents of first choice on the basis of strong evidence provided by major clinical trials evaluating hard renal endpoints that showed these drugs to slow the rate of renal function decline more effectively than other antihypertensive drug classes [8, 9]. In contrast, for patients with non-proteinuric CKD, earlier studies suggested that renin-angiotensin-aldosterone system (RAAS) inhibitors have no additional reno-protective benefits, whereas recent trials showed that dual blockade of RAAS is associated with elevated risk of acute renal failure and hyperkalemia [9–11]. With regards to the metabolic effects of antihypertensive agents, thiazide diuretics and conventional β-blockers were shown to reduce insulin sensitivity (IS) and to raise the risk of new-onset DM, whereas ACEIs and ARBs have rather neutral or even benefi-cial effects on metabolic profile [12–14]. This chapter aims to summarize how the presence of CKD and DM would influence the choice of antihypertensive treatment in patients with hypertension and HF, discussing currently available clinical evidence on the effects of antihypertensive treatment on renal endpoints and metabolic profile.

Choice of RAAS Inhibitors in Patients with Chronic Kidney Disease

Studies in Diabetic or Non-diabetic Proteinuric Kidney Disease

In the first clinical trial to evaluate the effect of RAAS block-ade on kidney disease progression, the Collaborative Study Group randomized 409 patients with type 1 DM and overt nephropathy (proteinuria >0.5 g/day and serum creatinine ≤2.5 mg/dl) to captopril or placebo [15]. After a median fol-low-up of 3 years, captopril treatment was associated with 43 % reduction in the risk of the primary end-point of doubling of serum creatinine, 50 % reduction in the composite outcomes of death, need for dialysis, and transplantation, and 30 % reduction in urinary albumin excretion (UAE) compared with the placebo. The slightly higher BP reduction evident in the captopril group during follow-up could not explain the differences in renal outcomes between the active treatment and placebo groups. Two subsequent large-scaled clinical trials explored the effects of RAAS inhibition on nephropathy progression in patients with type 2 DM [16, 17]. In the Reduction of Endpoints in NIDDM with the Angiotensin II Antagonist Losartan (RENAAL) study [16], 1,513 patients with type 2 DM and nephropathy [mean serum creatinine 1.9 mg/dl and median albumin-to-creatinine ratio (ACR) 1,237 mg/g] were randomly allocated to receive treatment with losartan (50–100 mg once daily) or placebo in addition to conventional antihypertensive therapy for a mean follow-up of 3.4 years. Treatment with losartan was associated with 16 % reduced risk of reaching the primary composite endpoint of doubling of serum creatinine, end-stage renal disease (ESRD) or death, as well as with 35 % decrease in ACR and 15 % reduction in the rate of renal function decline [16]. In the Irbesartan Diabetic Nephropathy Trial (IDNT) [17], 1,715 hypertensive patients with type 2 DM and overt nephropathy (UAE > 900 mg/day) were randomly assigned to receive treatment with irbesartan (300 mg/day), amlodipine (10 mg/day) or placebo for a mean follow-up of 2.6 years. Treatment with irbesartan induced a 20 % decrease relative to placebo and 23 % decrease relative to amlodipine in the primary composite endpoint consisting of time to occurrence of doubling of serum creatinine, ESRD or death from any cause; proteinuria was also reduced by 33 % with irbesartan versus 6 % with amlodipine and 10 % with placebo [17]. These beneficial effects of ACEIs and ARBs on slowing the progression of kidney injury in patients with diabetic nephropathy were also confirmed in subsequent carefully conducted meta-analyses [18, 19].

Post-hoc analyses of the trials mentioned above explored the association of baseline proteinuria and reductions in proteinuria throughout the study with the renal outcomes. In the

RENAAL trial, baseline proteinuria had a nearly linear relationship with the risk for the primary endpoint. Of note, for every 50 % reduction in albuminuria during the first 6 months, a 36 % risk reduction in the primary outcome and a 45 % reduction for the risk of ESRD at trial completion were evident. It was suggested that losartan could delay the need for renal replacement therapy or transplantation for 2 years and these renoprotective properties of losartan were mainly attributed to its anti-proteinuric effect and not to BP-lowering [20]. Similarly, in IDNT every twofold increase in baseline albuminuria was associated with doubled risk of the primary outcome. Regardless of treatment group, this risk was cut in half for every 50 % decrease in proteinuria at 1 year. Again, the greater renoprotective effect of irbesartan were attributed to its anti-proteinuric properties [21]. These findings provided a clear support to the significance of proteinuria as an intermediate endpoint in patients with overt diabetic nephropathy. The stage of CKD may represent another underlining factor that influences the benefit of RAAS inhibition. In the Collaborative Study patients with baseline serum creatinine >2.0 mg/dl achieved the greatest benefit from RAAS blockade; in particular, patients who received captopril had 74 % lower risk in the doubling of serum creatinine relative to placebo. In contrast, only a 4 % reduction in this endpoint was evident with ACE inhibition in patients with relatively preserved renal function (i.e., serum creatinine <1.0 mg/dl) [15].

Studies conducted in patients with non-diabetic kidney disease also support the beneficial impact of ACEIs on proteinuria reduction and delaying the progression of kidney injury. In the Ramipril-Efficacy-In-Nephropathy (REIN) 2 study, patients with mean serum creatinine of 2.4 mg/dL and urinary protein excretion >3 g/day were randomly assigned to receive treatment with ramipril (5 mg/day) or placebo on top of conventional BP-lowering therapy; ramipril induced significant reductions in proteinuria, the rate of renal function decline and in the risk of doubling of serum creatinine or progressing to ESRD relative to placebo, independently from changes in BP [22]. In the African American Study of Kidney Disease (AASK), 1,094 African-American patients with hypertensive kidney disease (estimated Glomerular Filtration Rate (eGFR): 20–65 ml/min/1.73 m^2 and mean proteinuria 0.6 g/day) were randomized to achieve goal mean arterial pressure 102–107 mmHg or ≤92 mmHg and to initial BP-lowering treatment with either metoprolol (2.5–10 mg/day), ramipril (2.5–10 mg/day) or amlodipine (5–10 mg/day) in a 3×2 factorial design. At trial end, patients treated with ramipril had a 36 % lower risk of reaching the composite renal endpoint of >50 % decrease in eGFR, ESRD or death relative to amlodipine, and also a 22 % reduced risk as compared to metoprolol.[23] A subsequent study randomized 224 patients with advanced stage non-diabetic kidney disease (SCr 3.1–5.0 mg/dl and mean proteinuria 1.6 g/day) to benazepril (20 mg/day) or placebo in addition to conventional antihypertensive treatment [24]. After an average follow-up of 3.4 years, benazepril was associated with 43 % reduced risk in reaching the primary outcome of doubling of serum creatinine, ESRD, or death as compared with placebo; further, benazepril decreased by 23 % the rate of eGFR decline and induced a 2.5-fold greater reduction in proteinuria than placebo. An earlier meta-analysis by Jafar et al. that included studies conducted in non-diabetic CKD patients, showed that antihypertensive regimens based on ACEIs were associated with 31 % lower risk in progression to ESRD and 30 % lower risk of the combined endpoint of doubling of serum creatinine or progression to ESRD [25].

Similarly to diabetic kidney disease, the reno-protective actions of RAAS inhibitors were shown to be more prominent in non-diabetic proteinuric nephropathies with higher levels of urinary protein excretion. In REIN-2, a higher degree of proteinuria at baseline was related to greater differences in the mean rate of GFR decline and in the proportion of patients reaching the primary outcome between the two groups, favoring the ACEI [22]. A post-hoc analysis of the AASK trial provided additional support to the important role of proteinuria reduction, showing that study participants who achieved an early reduction in proteinuria (i.e., at 6 months) experienced lower progression of their nephropathy to ESRD during 5 years [26]. Another earlier study that investigated the renoprotective properties of benazepril in patients with CKD of various causes also showed greater reductions in doubling of serum creatinine and need for dialysis in those with baseline proteinuria above 1 g/day [27]. The importance of the level of proteinuria is also supported by the aforementioned meta-analysis of Jafar et al.[28], in which ACEIs were shown to have similar renoprotective effects with other antihypertensive drug classes in CKD patients with urinary protein excretion lower than 0.5 g/day [25].

In addition to the above, a post-hoc analysis of data from the Losartan Intervention for Endpoint Reduction in Hypertension (LIFE) study [29] suggested that reduction in albuminuria during RAAS blockade was translated into cardiovascular risk reduction for patients with hypertension and left ventricle hypertrophy. The LIFE trial compared the effects of losartan versus atenolol on a primary composite endpoint of first occurrence of cardiovascular death, stroke or myocardial infraction during a mean follow-up period of 4.8 years. In this post-hoc analysis, when study participants were stratified according to the degree of albuminuria at baseline, it was shown that patients with the highest baseline UAE had a three- to fourfold greater risk of reaching the primary cardiovascular endpoint in comparison with those in the lowest UAE group. Further, the extent of albuminuria reduction at study completion was shown to be predictor of the decrease in the risk for the primary endpoint independently from the changes in BP levels [29].

As of this writing, there are no outcome data to support differences in renoprotective properties between ACEIs and ARBs in proteinuric kidney diseases. This was exemplified in the Diabetics Exposed to Telmisartan And enalapril (DETAIL) study, which compared the effects of enalapril and telmisartan in 250 hypertensive patients with type 2 DM and micro- or macro-albuminuria (UAE between 11 and 999 μg/min). After a mean follow-up of 2 years, both drugs exerted comparable effects on the rate of eGFR decline, albuminuria, BP, and the rates of progression to ESRD, cardiovascular events and all-cause mortality [30]. Some authors support the use of ARBs in place of ACEIs in the context of their better tolerability, lower incidence of hyperkalemia and cough, and the less frequent occurrence of the life-threatening complication of angioedema [31]. The higher cost of ARBs aggravates further this controversy surrounding this issue, but it has to be noted that ARBs have been proven to be cost-effective in the setting of diabetic nephropathy and in other clinical conditions [32] and generics for several ARB drugs are already available in many parts of the world. Overall, it seems reasonable to use the two classes interchangeably in patients with diabetic or non-diabetic proteinuria.

Studies in Non-proteinuric Kidney Disease

The reno-protective properties of RAAS inhibitors in diabetic or non-diabetic proteinuric kidney disease are strongly supported by solid background and clinical data; however, the question whether blockade of RAAS has similar beneficial effects on patients with hypertension and early stage CKD or in subjects with impaired renal function and non-proteinuric nephropathy remains largely unanswered in the context of the absence of randomized clinical studies investigating specifically the effects of ACEIs and ARBs on hard renal outcomes in these patient populations. This issue is of major clinical significance, as with the current definition of CKD, it is estimated that about 40 % of the adult population aged >70 years have eGFR < 60 ml/min/1.73 m², whereas only 5 % have macro-albuminuria. Among patients with hypertension, about 15 % have impaired renal function (ranging up to 30 % in those aged >65 years), but again less than 5 % of hypertensive CKD individuals have macro-albuminuria [33, 34]. A major systematic review on this field suggested that guidelines on the administration of RAAS blockers towards reno-protection have limited relevance to patients >70 years of age; most of the studies on which contemporary guidelines were based did not enrol patients of this age group at all, with the exception of one trial [the Antihypertensive and Lipid Lowering Treatment to Prevent Heart Attack Trial (ALLHAT)], which recruited an important number of elderly individuals [34]. In recent years, however, data on reno-protection on this patient population were brought to light from secondary analyses of major cardiovascular outcome trials.

A previous meta-analysis [35] loudly challenged the beneficial effects of RAAS blockers on delaying kidney disease progression. In studies comparing ACEIs or ARBs with the placebo, blockade of RAAS improved all renal endpoints, but this effect was accompanied by more pronounced BP lowering in active treatment groups. Studies that compared ACEIs or ARBs with other antihypertensive drug classes showed a relative risk (RR) reduction of 29 % (RR: 0.71; 95 %CI 0.49–1.04) for doubling of serum creatinine and a slight significant benefit on incidence of ESRD (RR: 0.87; 95 %CI 0.75–0.99). Among studies enrolling only diabetics, those that compared ACEIs and ARBs with placebo showed RAAS blockers to be associated with significant reductions of 21 and 22 % in the risk of ESRD and doubling of serum creatinine, respectively; however, studies in diabetic individuals comparing RAAS inhibitors with active treatment yielded no renal benefit of RAAS blockade [35]. It has to be noted that this meta-analysis met important criticism for several methodological issues, i.e. presence of substantial heterogeneity across studies included in analysis, domination by ALLHAT on the pooled outcome estimates, no evaluation of the potential impact of proteinuria and CKD stage, equal attention to intermediate and hard renal outcomes, absence of patient-level data, and performance of separate analysis of placebo-controlled and active treatment-controlled studies, despite the fact that in studies using placebo as a comparator patients were administered background antihypertensive treatment [36–38]. As ALLHAT trial substantially influenced the pooled estimates (discussed below) [39], this meta-analysis seemed to aggregate patients with true diabetic nephropathy and diabetic patients with other forms of kidney injury (i.e. ischemic nephropathy) [37] and ALLHAT domination may have overridden any impact in patients with diabetic nephropathy. In this context, these findings were not considered strong enough to controvert the solid and consistent results of studies on RAAS inhibition in patients with diabetic or non-diabetic proteinuric kidney disease; however, this meta-analysis raised for the first-time the issue of renoprotection in patients with non-advanced CKD or non-proteinuric CKD.

The first trial with population like the above was the Appropriate Blood Pressure Control in Diabetes (ABCD) [40], that included 470 hypertensive subjects with type 2 DM, of whom only 18 % had macro-albuminuria. Baseline creatinine clearance (CrCl) was about 85 ml/min/1.73 m^2 overall and 75 ml/min/1.73 m^2 in the subgroup of patients with macro-albuminuria. Participants were randomized to nisoldipine or enalapril and intensive or moderate BP control in a 2×2 factorial design. There was no difference in CrCl between the two groups over 5.3 years of follow-up, although enalapril significantly lowered UAE. However, the most definite end-point of incident ESRD was not recorded. Furthermore, it is unknown whether this benefit of enalapril on proteinuria would translate into retardation of renal disease if the follow-up was extended.

ALLHAT randomised >33,000 patients aged >55 years with hypertension and at least one more cardiovascular risk factor to chlorthalidone, amlodipine and lisinopril with a primary cardiovascular outcome. As patients with serum creatinine >2.0 mg/dL and patients treated with an ACEI for underlying CKD were excluded from the study by protocol, the average eGFR of study participants at baseline was 78 ml/min/1.73 m^2. This study did include measurements of urine protein excretion, but on the basis of the aforementioned exclusion criteria, participants with proteinuria should have been a minority. At the end of the study, eGFR was significantly higher in amlodipine than chlorthalidone, and lisinopril groups (75 versus 70 and 71 ml/min/1.73 m^2 respectively). In post-hoc analysis, there were no differences in the incidence of ESRD or a $\geq$50 % decrement in eGFR between the three groups in the whole study cohort and in sub-groups of patients with mild (60–89 mL/min/1.73 m^2) or moderate-severe (<60 mL/min/1.73 m^2) reduction of baseline GFR [39]. These results are in direct contrast with the afore-mentioned findings of the IDNT, where amlodipine resulted in worsened renal function decline; this, however, is rather directly related to different characteristics of the populations under study [38]. The authors of ALLHAT suggested that presumably participants with decreased eGFR were patients with ischemic nephropathy, for which an overwhelming reno-protective effect of ACEIs is not expected [39]. Absence of renoprotective effects of lisinopril and (possibly beneficial actions of amlodipine) in a population with mean age 67 years and mean eGFR 78 ml/min/1.73 m^2, with the few indi-viduals at risk for CKD progression suffering mainly from ischemic renal disease seems by all means reasonable.

Additional support to the aforementioned findings is pro-vided by the renal outcomes of another cardiovascular trial, the Avoiding Cardiovascular Events through Combination Therapy in Patients Living with Systolic Hypertension (ACCOMPLISH). In this study, 11,506 hypertensive patients with high cardiovascular risk profile were randomly allocated to receive benazepril plus amlodipine or benazepril plus hydrochlorothiazide combinations. ACCOMPLISH trial was terminated earlier than the prespecified follow-up duration due to benefit of the benazepril plus amlodipine combination in the primary cardiovascular endpoint. With regards to the characteristics of the population studied, about 85 % were aged >65 years and 60 % had DM; however, the mean eGFR of study participants at baseline was 79 mL/min/1.73 m^2, 19 % of patients had micro-albuminuria, 5 % had macro-albuminuria and about 10 % of the patients had eGFR <60 mL/min/1.73 m^2 [41]. The ACCOMPLISH trial showed that the benazepril plus amlodipine combination produced a slower annual rate of eGFR decrease than the benazepril plus hydrochlorothiazide combination (−0.88 versus −4.22 mL/min/1.73 m^2 per year), despite the less effective reduction in albuminuria [41]. Furthermore, the benazepril plus amlodipine combination was shown to be associated with a 48 % reduction in the composite renal endpoints of doubling of serum creatinine, eGFR < 15 mL/min/1.73 m^2 and dialysis (HR 0.52; 95 %CI 0.41–0.65) and 27 % reduction in doubling of serum creatinine, ESRD and death (HR 0.73; 95 %CI 0.64–0.84). The slower kidney disease progression with the addition of a dihydropyridine to a RAAS inhibitor versus a thiazide diuretic does not represent an unexpected finding in groups of patients with mean age >65 years and preserved renal function (mean eGFR well above 60 ml/min/1.73 m^2). Further, absence of an anti-proteinuric impact of the dihydropiridine reasonably did not influence the occurrence of hard renal endpoints in the ACCOMPLISH trial, as elderly patients with preserved renal function and normo-albuminuria are more likely to suffer GFR reduction through pre-renal acute renal failure (i.e. from dehydration and hypotension) than through proteinuric injury.

High Doses of RAAS-Inhibitors or Dual RAAS Blockade

Although several research efforts were made over the past years in order to develop novel treatment strategies targeting on delaying the progression of proteinuric kidney diseases, none of them was approved for implementation in daily clinical practice. In this context, several investigators have evaluated the potential benefits of aggressive RAAS inhibition towards reno-protection [38]. In this direction, evidence derived from short-term randomized clinical studies including patients with micro- or macroalbuminuria have suggested that administration of a single RAAS inhibitor in ultra-high dose (i.e. two to three times the maximum dose recommended for treatment of hypertension) could have a more potent anti-proteinuric effect than conventional doses, without causing serious complications [42–45]. Other studies showed that dual blockade of RAAS with combination of ACEIs and ARBs was associated with more effective reduction in albuminuria than single blockade at maximum recommended doses [46, 47]. These findings were supported by the results of the Combination Treatment of ARB and ACEI in Non diabetic Renal Disease (COOPERATE) trial, which showed that the combined administration of trandolapril and losartan in subjects with non-diabetic proteinuric kidney disease led to 60 % decrease in doubling of serum creatinine or incidence of ESRD relative to mono-therapy with either drug alone [48]. These results were initially considered perfectly reasonable and on this basis, dual RAAS blockade was implemented in daily clinical practice as an additional therapeutic option towards reno-protection for patients with proteinuric nephropathies; however, the above-mentioned findings were followed by great embarrassment for the international nephrology community when the whole trial was proven to be a fraud [49].

The effects of double RAAS blockade with ACEI/ARB combination on hard cardiovascular and renal endpoints were investigated in the Ongoing Telmisartan Alone and in combination with Ramipril Global Endpoint Trial (ONTARGET) [50] (Table 3.1). In this study, 23,400 patients with history of a previous cardiovascular event were randomized to receive treatment with ramipril 10 mg daily, telmisartan 80 mg daily, or their combination for a median follow-up period of 56 months. This trial was expected to provide the definite answer on the potential role of combined RAAS inhibition as an alternative treatment approach for cardiovascular and renal risk reduction. Indeed, the ONTARGET trial provided important information with regards to the harmful renal effects of dual RAAS blockade in patients with cardiovascular disease, but left unresolved the issue of the potential benefits of this treatment approach in patients with proteinuric nephropathies due to the characteristics of the population studied; 68 % of the patients participating in the ONTARGET trial were hypertensives, 37 % diabetic, and

Table 3.1 Outcome trial evaluating the effects of dual RAAS inhibition on cardiovascular and renal end-points

	ONTARGET	ALTITUDE	VA NEPHRON-D
N	25,620	8,561	1,448
Study groups	Ramipril 10 mg, Telmisartan 80 mg, combination of both	Aliskiren 300 mg versus placebo on top of ACEI or ARB	Lisinopril 10–40 mg versus placebo on top of losartan 100 mg
Primary composite end-point	Death from cardiovascular causes, myocardial infarction, stroke, or hospitalization for HF	Cardiovascular death or first occurrence of cardiac arrest with resuscitation; myocardial infarction; stroke; unplanned hospitalization for HF; ESRD, death attributable to kidney failure, or need for RRT with no dialysis or transplantation available or initiated; or doubling of serum creatinine	First occurrence of a change in the estimated GFR (a decline of ≥30 ml/min/1.73 m² if the initial estimated GFR was ≥60 ml/min/1.73 m² or a decline of ≥50 % if the initial estimated GFR was <60 ml/min/1.73 m²), ESRD, or death
Secondary renal composite end-point	Any dialysis, doubling of serum creatinine, or death	ESRD, death attributable to renal failure, or the need for RRT with no dialysis or transplantation available or initiated; or doubling of serum creatinine	First occurrence of a decline in the estimated GFR or ESRD

Follow-up (years)	4.7	2.8	2.2
Population characteristics			
Age (years)	66.4	64.5	64.6
Gender (Male/Female, %)	73/27	68/32	99/1
BMI (kg/m²)	28.1	29.9	34.6
Hypertension (%)	69	94.5	100
Diabetes (%)	37	100	100
Mean baseline BP (mmHg)	142/82	137/74	137/73
Baseline estimated GFR (ml/min/1.73 m²)	73.6	57	53.7

(continued)

Table 3.1 (continued)

	ONTARGET	ALTITUDE	VA NEPHRON-D
Estimated GFR <60 ml/min/1.73 m^2 (%)	24	67.5	62
Urinary albumin excretion			
Normo-albuminuria (%)	82.9	14.5	0
Micro-albuminuria (%)	13.1	25.6	0
Macro-albuminuria (%)	4	58.4	100

| Main findings | Primary composite outcome: telmisartan was not inferior to ramipril; combination treatment was not superior to ramipril, and was associated with higher incidence of hypotension, hyperkalemia, and syncope. Renal outcomes: telmisartan had similar effects with ramipril; combination treatment increased by 2.2-fold the risk of dialysis for acute kidney failure compared with ramipril | Terminated early because of hypotension, hyperkalemia, and acute kidney failure in the aliskiren group

Cardiovascular composite: 11 % increase with aliskiren (HR 1.11; CI: 0.99–1.25, P = 0.09), driven by 2.4-fold higher risk of resuscitated cardiac arrest

Renal composite: no difference between groups (HR 1.03; 95 % CI: 0.87–1.23, P = 0.74) | Terminated early due to elevated risk of hyperkalemia and acute kidney failure in the combination group

Primary composite renal endpoint: no difference between the combination and mono-therapy groups (HR: 0.88; 95 % CI: 0.70–1.12, P = 0.30) |

Abbreviations: ACEI angiotensin converting enzyme inhibitor, *ALTITUDE* Aliskiren Trial in Type 2 Diabetes Using Cardiorenal Endpoints, *ARB* angiotensin receptor blocker, *BMI* body mass index, *BP* blood pressure, *CI* confidence interval, *GFR* glomerular filtration rate, *ESRD* end-stage renal disease, *HF* heart failure, *HR* hazard ratio, *ONTARGET* Ongoing Telmisartan Alone and in combination with Ramipril Global Endpoint Trial, *RAAS* renin angiotensin aldosterone system, *RRT* renal replacement therapy, *VA NEPHRON-D* The Veterans Affairs Nephropathy in Diabetes study

23 % had CKD, defined as eGFR below 60 ml/min/1.73 m^2, but only 13 % had micro-albuminuria and around 3 % macro-albuminuria and overt diabetic nephropathy. This study showed that patients who were assigned to receive dual RAAS blockade had 24 % higher risk of dialysis or doubling of serum creatinine relative to those who received ramipril alone (HR 1.24; 95 %CI 1.01–1.51) [50]. Further, albuminuria exhibited a temporal increasing trend during follow-up in all three study groups, with the combination treatment display-ing the lowest rate of UAE rise. These findings were consid-ered by several investigators as conclusive evidence against the administration of combined RAAS inhibition in patients with CKD; other investigators also challenged the value of proteinuria as predictor of kidney disease progression. It has to be noted, however, that such conclusions cannot be drawn from a study cohort, in which the vast majority of participants were normo-albuminuric at baseline. A more careful glance at renal outcomes of the ONTARGET trial indicates that the difference in the occurrence of primary renal endpoint dur-ing follow-up between study groups was arisen from signifi-cant differences only in dialysis for acute renal failure, whereas the risks of doubling of serum creatinine and dialysis due to incident ESRD were similar between groups. A potential explanation for this finding could be the more fre-quent occurrence of hypotension and acute renal failure in patients receiving dual RAAS inhibition. Thus, these findings represent another characteristic example of the harmful renal effects of aggressive RAAS blockade in predisposed patients (i.e., elderly normotensive patients with impaired renal function, most probably attributed to ischemic renal disease) [51, 52].

Another tool in our therapeutic armamentarium that was suggested to offer additional benefits towards reno-protection is the blockage of RAAS with the recently introduced direct renin inhibitor aliskiren. The effects of aliskiren on protein-uria were evaluated in the Aliskiren in the Evaluation of Proteinuria in Diabetes (AVOID) study, in which 599 patients with type 2 DM, hypertension and macro-albuminuria were randomly allocated to aliskiren (150 mg force-titrated to 300 mg daily) or placebo on top of losartan 100 mg and optimal BP-lowering therapy. After a mean follow-up of 6 months, addition of aliskiren to losartan along with standard antihypertensive therapy was associated with a 20 % higher decrease in ACR relative to placebo [53]; of note, these anti-proteinuric properties of aliskiren were shown to be independent from BP reduction [54].

On the basis of this beneficial impact of aliskiren on proteinuria in the AVOID study, the subsequent Aliskiren Trial in Type 2 Diabetes Using Cardiorenal Endpoints (ALTITUDE) trial evaluated the effect of adding aliskiren 300 mg daily relative to placebo on top of standard therapy with ACEI or ARB on a primary composite cardio-renal endpoint consisting of the time to cardiovascular death or a first occurrence of cardiac arrest with resuscitation, non-fatal myocardial infarction, nonfatal stroke, unplanned hospitalization for HF, ESRD, death attributable to CKD, or the need for renal-replacement therapy, or doubling of the baseline serum creatinine. ALTITUDE was prematurely stopped after the second interim efficacy analysis because of frequent occurrence of renal adverse events, hyperkalemia and hypotension in the aliskiren group [55]; this early termination of the ALTITUDE trial gained the great attention of the international nephrology community and was considered again as the end of dual RAAS inhibition. The publication of the full-report of the trial shed light on several issues [11]. All components of primary composite cardio-renal outcome of the ALTITUDE did not significantly differ between the aliskiren and placebo groups, with the exception of resuscitated cardiac arrest. With regards to the renal components of the primary outcome, events of doubling of serum creatinine were evenly distributed between groups, whereas the endpoints of ESRD, dialysis or death due to renal failure were also not significantly different. Moreover, a greater reduction by 1.3/0.6 mmHg in BP and a more effective decrease in ACR by 14 % was noted in the aliskiren relative to the placebo group. In contrast, the main differences noted between groups were the proportion of study participants with hyperkalemia (11.2 % vs. 7.2 %), and reported hypotension (12.1 % vs. 8.3 %) (P<0.001 for both) [11].

A plausible explanation for the early termination of the ALTITUDE trial due to renal complications can be provided again by the careful evaluation of the characteristics of the population enrolled in the study (Table 3.1). Following the inclusion criteria of macro-albuminuria or eGFR 30–60 ml/min/1.73 m^2 and micro-albuminuria or eGFR 30–60 ml/min/1.73 m^2 and history of cardiovascular events, the study cohort of ALTITUDE was closer to that of cardiovascular and not renal outcome trials; further, the population characteristics of the ALTITUDE trial differed significantly from that of AVOID. In particular, the mean age of the ALTITUDE population was 65 years, 42 % had cardiovascular disease, 67 % had eGFR lower than 45 ml/min/1.73 m^2, and only 58 % of patients were macro-albuminuric. Enrolled patients also had BP lower than 135/85 mmHg, or BP between 135/85 and 170/110 mmHg at first visits if treated with at least three BP-lowering agents; thus mean baseline BP was 137/74 mmHg and 69 % of participants were already taking diuretics in combination with ACEI or ARB. On this basis, a high proportion of patients were particularly prediposed to complications from aggressive BP reduction (indeed hypotension was more frequently recorded in elderly individuals and in patients treated with loop diuretics). Therefore, the serious renal complications that resulted in premature termination of the ALTITUDE trial can be directly attributed to aggressive RAAS blocking in susceptible individuals. In this context, ALTITUDE resembled ONTARGET in showing that double RAAS blockade may provide more harm than good in predisposed individuals with CKD [56].

Finally, efficacy and tolerability of dual RAAS inhibition for proteinuric nephropathy was also evaluated in the recently published Veterans Affairs Nephropathy in Diabetes (VA NEPHRON-D) study [10], in which 1,448 patients with type 2 DM, macro-albuminuria and eGFR ranging from 30 to 89.9 ml/min/1.73 m^2 were randomly assigned to receive lisinospril (10–40 mg daily) or placebo on top of treatment with the ARB losartan at a dose of 100 mg per day. The primary composite renal endpoint of the study was the first occurrence of a change in eGFR (a decline of $\geq$30 ml/min/1.73 m^2 if the baseline eGFR was $\geq$60 ml/min/1.73 m^2 or a decline of $\geq$50 % if the baseline eGFR was <60 ml/min/1.73 m^2), ESRD, or death. VA NEPHRON-D study was also prematurely terminated at a median follow-up period of 2.2 years due to safety concerns, as combined RAAS blockade elevated the risk of hyperkalemia in comparison with mono-therapy (6.3 vs 2.6 events per 100 person-years, P<0.001), as well as the risk of acute renal failure (12.2 vs 6.7 events per 100 person-years, P<0.001). The risk of the primary renal endpoint did not significantly differ between groups in the whole study cohort (HR with the combination therapy: 0.88; 95 % CI: 0.70–1.12, P=0.30) and among pre-specified sub-groups (P>0.10 for all interactions). With regards to the secondary endpoint of decline in eGFR or ESRD, a trend towards a benefit of the combination therapy was noted after about 6–12 months of treatment, but this effect was not sustained with longer follow-up (HR: 0.78; 95 % CI: 0.58–1.05, P=0.10) [10].

The early termination of VA NEPHRON-D trial due to heightened risk of acute renal failure and hyperkalemia should be rather considered the definite end of dual RAAS blockade for renoprotection. This is mostly because VA NEPHRON-D trial included a relevant population, i.e. patients with diabetic nephropathy and macro-albuminuria, with a mean age of 64.5 years, of whom 23 % had coronary artery disease, 16 % had congestive HF and 30 % had eGFR lower than 45 ml/min/1.73 m^2, whereas mean baseline BP of study participants was 137/73 mmHg with background treatment with 3 or more BP-lowering agents [10] (Table 3.1). Overall, as HF with decreased cardiac-output is a typical predisposing factor for acute renal failure, it seems reasonable to avoid dual ACEI/ARB combination for renoprotection in these patients. It may be argued by some that a benefit of dual blockade in retarding proteinuric CKD progression could be still present in healthier populations with little risk for acute renal failure with aggressive RAAS blocking (i.e., young individuals with proteinuric kidney disease, preserved renal function, absence of overt vascular disease and high-adherence to low dietary potassium intake). As specific treatments against proteinuric kidney disease are still lacking a study on such a population may appear in the future, but any results should be cautiously interpreted.

As in heart failure patients, combining an aldosterone-receptor-antagonist with ACEIs or ARBs is proposed as another treatment option for slowing kidney disease progression, since plasma aldosterone is increased in CKD and may independently promote renal damage [57]; further, blockade of RAAS with the use of ACEIs or ARBs does not necessarily lead to prolonged lowering in plasma aldosterone levels [58]. Several pilot studies in proteinuric CKD have revealed promising results that addition of spironolactone in patients with proteinuria already treated with ACEIs or ARBs provides an additional anti-proteinuric effect to that exerted by mono-therapy [59–62]. In parallel, administration of eplerenone in addition to standard antihypertensive treatment with an ACEI was associated with further reduction in UAE in patients with hypertension and left ventricular hypertrophy [63]. In a more recent study 81 patients with DM, hypertension, and macro-albuminuria already under treatment with lisinopril 80 mg were randomized to losartan 100 mg, spironolactone 25 mg or placebo [64]. After 48 weeks of follow-up, ACR was significantly reduced by 34 % in the spironolactone group and by 16.8 % in the losartan group as compared to placebo; ambulatory BP, CrCl, sodium and protein intake, and glycemic control did not significantly differ between groups. However, addition of sprironolactone and losartan to lisinopril resulted in elevated serum potassium levels (yet on average <5.2 meq/L in all groups). Use of low-dose spironolactone in addition to ACEIs or ARBs seems to be a promising treatment approach for proteinuric patients, but large outcome trials evaluating hard renal end-points should be performed before any treatment recommendations can be made. This is mostly due to the concern of heightened rates of hyperkalemia [65], as was also exemplified by large population studies [66] following the extended use of spironolactone for HF after the publication of the Randomized Aldactone Evaluation Study (RALES) [67].

Choice of Antihypertensive Treatment in Patients with Diabetes Mellitus

For more than two decades one of the most active area of research topics in the field of hypertension therapeutics was the possible effects of major antihypertensive drug classes on carbohydrate metabolism and the development of new-onset DM [14]. In this regard, numerous clinical studies have investigated the impact of antihypertensive agents on insulin sensitivity (IS) and glycemic control, whereas large outcome trials have explored the potential association between antihypertensive agents and incident DM. Another important issue is the possible harmful impact of antihypertensive therapy – related new-onset DM on cardiovascular outcomes [14]; thus, presence of DM should be taken into consideration in the choice of the appropriate BP-lowering therapy in patients with hypertension and HF.

Effects of Antihypertensive Agents on Insulin Sensitivity

Preliminary reports from older studies suggested that thiazide and loop diuretics (especially in higher doses, i.e. equivalent to ≥25 mg of hydrochlorothiazide) and conventional β-blockers deteriorate IS and glycemic control and elevate the risk of developing new-onset DM [68–73]. Data on β-blockers and their metabolic effects gain much more interest, as newer, vasodilating agents were proposed to have a much different metabolic profile than conventional ones [74]. As β-blockers remain first-line treatment for HF, these effects are of major importance when selecting the appropriate agents in these patients. In this regard, initial studies that compared the metabolic effect of a vasodilating β-blocker carvedilol with either metoprolol [75–77] or atenolol [78, 79] in patients with hypertension or hypertension and DM showed significant differences between groups, as treatment with conventional β-blockers resulted in reduced IS. This favorable effect was strongly supported by the results of the large Glycemic Effects in Diabetes Mellitus: Carvedilol-Metoprolol Comparison in Hypertensives (GEMINI) multi-center trial that compared effects of carvedilol to metoprolol treatment on IS in 1,235 hypertensive patients with type 2 DM already treated with an ACEI or an ARB. This study revealed a significant reduction in the Homeostasis Model Assessment-Insulin Resistance (HOMA-IR) index of about 9 % with carvedilol relative to metoprolol [77]. Nebivolol, another β_1-blocker that has been reported to increase nitric oxide (NO) production from endothelium, thus resulting in peripheral vasodilatation [80], was not previously shown to significantly affect IS in patients with hypertension [79] and/ or type 2 DM [81, 82]. These beneficial metabolic effects of nebivolol were confirmed in recent studies that showed improvement in glucose metabolism with nebivolol relative to metoprolol in patients with metabolic syndrome [83].

Studies evaluating the effects of ACEIs on metabolic profile suggest that use of these agents in hypertensive patients improves, or at least, does not deteriorate IS. Acute oral administration of 25 mg of captopril during euglycemic hyperinsulinemic clamp in patients with type 2 DM was shown to be associated with a significant increase in insulin-induced glucose disposal [84]. Similarly, subsequent studies with captopril, enalapril, cilazapril, and fosinopril showed improvement in IS and glycemic control in patients with hypertension and/or type 2 DM [69, 85, 86], whereas in other cases treatment with ACEIs was shown to have no impact on these parameters [82, 87, 88], suggesting that this antihypertensive drug class has a positive, or at least neutral effect on metabolic profile.

Similarly to ACEIs, the currently available data on the use of ARBs suggest that these agents may have a neutral or positive impact on IS. A beneficial metabolic effect is particularly applied to telmisartan, that has been proposed to exert unique insulin-sensitizing properties [89]. This is in relation to the fact that telmisartan was shown to activate the peroxisome proliferator-activated receptor (PPAR)–γ receptors, an action that was not proven for other ARBs [90]. Activation of the PPAR–γ receptors is well-documented that results in IS improvement, as it represents the main mechanism of action for thiazolidinendiones [91]. In a randomized study including patients with hypertension and impaired glucose tolerance or type 2 DM, treatment with telmisartan was associated with a 26 % decrease in the HOMA-IR index along with 8 % reduction in fasting glucose, 9 % lowering in HbA1c, and 10 % decrease in fasting insulin, in contrast to losartan, that had no influence on any of these parameters [92]. A mild beneficial effect of telmisartan on HOMA-IR index is also supported by subsequent clinical studies [93–95]. Furthermore, treatment with candesartan was also related to a significant decrease of about 25 % in insulin resistance [96]. It has to be noted, however, that the potentially beneficial effects of ARBs on metabolic profile have to be confirmed in larger studies including euglycemic hyperinsulinemic clamp measurements.

Effects of Antihypertensive Agents on New-Onset DM

Data from Hypertension Outcome Trials Evaluating New-Onset DM as a Secondary Outcome

During the previous 15 years, a number of large-scaled outcome trials attempted to investigate as a secondary outcome, the effect of various antihypertensive drug classes on the occurrence of new-onset DM. Most of these studies compared newer (i.e. ACEIs, ARBs, or calcium channel blockers, or combinations of those) with conventional antihypertensive regimens (i.e. thiazide diuretics or β-blockers or combinations). In the Captopril Prevention Project (CAPPP) trial, in which above 11,000 patients with hypertension were randomly assigned to captopril or conventional treatment with diuretics, β-blockers or both, captopril-based regimen was shown to be associated with significantly lower incidence of type 2 DM in comparison with the conventional regimen (14 % lower RR in the intention-to-treat and 21 % in the on-treatment analyses respectively) [97]. The Intervention as a Goal in Hypertension Treatment (INSIGHT) study randomized more than 6,000 hypertensive individuals to a regimen based on long-acting nifedipine or co-amilozide (hydrochlorothiazide plus amiloride) [98]. After a mean follow-up of about 4 years, the occurrence of new-onset DM was lower in patients receiving nifedipine than in those receiving diuretic-based treatment (4.3 % versus 5.6 %). The LIFE study randomized 9,193 patients with hypertension and left ventricular hypertrophy to receive treatment with losartan-based or atenolol-based antihypertensive regimen for at least 4 years. Among patients without DM at trial initiation, those who were randomized to the losartan-based regimen had an 25 % lower risk of developing new-onset DM throughout the study compared to those on atenolol-based treatment [99].

One of the largest outcome trials in hypertension to evaluate the impact of various antihypertensive drug classes on the incidence of new-onset DM was the ALLHAT trial, in which more than 33,000 hypertensive patients were randomly assigned to a chlorothalidone-based, an amlodipine-based or a lisinopril-based therapy, as discussed above. Among non-diabetic patients at baseline, chlorothalidone treatment was associated with significantly higher incidence of new-onset DM during the 4 years of follow-up than treatment with either amlodipine or lisinopril (11.8 % versus 9.8 % and 8.1 % respectively) [100]. In the Second Australian National Blood Pressure Study (ANBP2), above 6,000 patients aged 65–84 years were randomized to receive treatment with an ACEI (mainly enalapril) or a diuretic (mainly hydrochlorothiazide) [101]. After a median follow-up of 4.1 years, treatment with the ACEI-based regimen resulted in 31 % lower risk of developing new-onset DM compared to the diuretic-based regimen (DM incidence of 4.54 % vs 6.58 % respectively) [102]. The International Verapamil-Trandorapril Study (INVEST) randomized 22,576 hypertensive patients with coronary artery disease to receive verapamil-based or atenolol-based antihypertensive treatment. Again, non-diabetic patients at entry in the verapamil group had a 15 % lower risk of developing new-onset DM than subjects in the atenolol group after a median follow-up of 2.7 years [103]. In agreement with the findings of the INVEST trial, the Anglo-Scandinavian Cardiac Outcomes Trial (ASCOT), which assigned more than 19,000 hypertensive patients to an amlodipine plus perindopril arm or an atenolol plus bendro-flumethiazide arm, showed that the incidence of new-onset DM was 30 % lower in the amlodipine than in the atenolol group after a median follow-up of 5.5 years [104].

In addition to the above, effects of antihypertensive agents on incidence of new-onset DM were investigated in other trials using placebo as a comparator. In the Heart Outcomes Prevention Evaluation (HOPE) trial, a total of 9,297 patients with an age above 55 years were randomly assigned to receive ramipril (10 mg daily) or placebo on top of their standard medication, which included other antihypertensive agents, for a mean observational period of 5 years. At trial completion, treatment with ramipril induced a 34 % reduction in the incidence of new-onset DM relative to placebo in originally non-diabetic study participants [105]. The Candesartan in Heart Failure Assessment of Reduction in Mortality and morbidity (CHARM) trial, (which had as main inclusion criterion symptomatic HF and not hypertension) revealed that treatment with the ARB candesartan resulted in a significant decrease of 19 % in the risk of new-onset DM as compared with placebo [106].

It has to be noted, however, that some studies did not show statistically significant elevation in the risk of new-onset DM with conventional or significant reductions with newer antihypertensive agents. In the Systolic Hypertension in the Elderly Program (SHEP) trial, patients with isolated systolic hypertension and above 60 years of age were randomized to stepped-care therapy with 12.5–25.0 mg per day of chlorthalidone or matching placebo aiming to reach goal BP (systolic BP <160 mmHg). When BP remained above the goal, study investigators were permitted by protocol to add atenolol or reserpine; thus, 32 % of patients randomly allocated to receive chlorthalidone were also administered atenolol [107]. After 4.5 years of follow-up, incidence of DM was slightly higher in the chlorthalidone group compared with the placebo (8.6 % vs 7.5 %) [107], a finding that was translated into a non-significant 20 % elevation in the risk of new-onset DM (RR: 1.2; 95 % CI: 0.9–1.5) with this treatment [108]. The Swedish Trial in Old Patients with Hypertension 2 (STOP-Hypertension 2) study, in which 6,614 elderly hypertensive patients were randomly allocated to conventional treatment (β-blockers or diuretics) or to either ACEI-based or calcium channel blocker (CCB)-based regimen, also reported negative results; along with the absence of significant difference in the composite primary cardiovascular outcome, no significant differences in incidence of new-onset DM between the three study groups were evident after about 4.5 years of follow-up [109]. In addition, the Nordic Diltiazem (NORDIL) study, in which 10,881 hypertensive patients were randomized to diltiazem, or diuretics and β-blockers, or both, a 13 % lower risk of developing new-onset DM was evident in the diltiazem group, but this difference did not reach statistical significance [110]. The Study on Cognition and Prognosis in the Elderly (SCOPE), conducted in about 5,000 elderly hypertensive subjects aged 70–89 years, showed also a non-significant decrease of 19 % in incidence of new-onset DM with candesartan relative to placebo [111].

The only hypertension outcome trial that compared the treatment effects of thiazide diuretics against that of β-blockers on incidence of new-onset DM was the Heart Attack Primary Prevention in Hypertension (HAPPHY) trial, published almost 25 years ago. In this trial, above 6,500 men aged 40–64 years with mild to moderate hypertension were randomized to receive a thiazide diuretic or a β-blocker. As exactly happened with all components of the composite primary endpoint, incidence of new-onset DM did not significantly differ between groups after 45 months of treatment [112]. Similarly, only one outcome trial provided a direct head-to-head comparison of the effect of agents from two newer antihypertensive classes; the Valsartan Antihypertensive Long-term Use Evaluation (VALUE) study randomized more than 15,000 hypertensive patients to the ARB valsartan or the CCB amlodipine for a mean follow-up period of 4.2 years [113]. Although no significant difference in the primary composite outcome between the two drugs was noted, treatment with valsartan resulted in a 23 % lower risk of new-onset DM in comparison with amlodipine [114].

Overall, the majority of the above mentioned randomized studies support a beneficial impact of newer (ACEIs, ARBs and CCBs) over older (diuretics, β-blockers) antihypertensive agents on the incidence of new-onset DM; it has to be noted, however, that these studies suffer from some methodological limitation that may affect the strength of their findings and thus, the conclusions that can be drawn from them. First, none of the aforementioned studies published so far reporting effects of antihypertensive treatment on new-onset DM had the incidence of DM as the primary trial endpoint [97–99, 101, 103, 104, 107–110, 113]. Second, in some of these studies an ACEI [97, 109] or a CCB [109, 110] was compared to conventional treatment consisting of either diuretics or β-blockers or their combination, and therefore an individual treatment effect of the later antihypertensive classes cannot be easily evaluated. In some studies, a great proportion of patients in the various arms were receiving background treatment with second-line antihypertensive agents that could also affect IS and glycemic control towards the same [101, 103, 104, 110] or the opposite direction [101, 103, 110–112], making again difficult the assessment of the net impact of the main agents on the incidence of DM. Further, the possibility of detection bias in those of the above studies that were open-label with blinded end-point assessment can not be excluded [97, 101, 103, 109, 110, 112], as DM may have been more intensively sought in patients receiving conventional treatment. In other cases, new-onset DM was not diagnosed with the most accurate methods, i.e. it was self reported [105]. Finally, in trials comparing active antihypertensive regimens, the observed differences [97–101, 103, 104] could be arisen either from a harmful effect of conventional agents or from a beneficial impact of the newer drugs, a fact not allowing firm conclusions to be drawn.

Data from Trials and Meta-analyses Investigating the Effects of Antihypertensive Agents on Metabolic Parameters and New-Onset DM

The impact of antihypertensive therapy on new-onset DM was also explored in clinical studies that specifically aimed to evaluate the effects of such drugs on the metabolic profile. In the Antihypertensive Treatment and Lipid Profile in a North of Sweden Efficacy Evaluation (ALPINE) study, 392 subjects with hypertension were randomly assigned to receive treatment with low-dose hydrochlorothiazide alone or combined with atenolol or treatment with the ARB candesartan alone or combined with felodipine. This study showed that treatment for 12 months with the diuretic-based regimen resulted in elevation of fasting plasma glucose and insulin, whereas no increase in these parameters was evident in patients who received candesartan; further, hydrochlorothiazide treatment was associated with significantly higher incidence of new-onset DM than treatment with the ARB candesartan (4.1 % vs 0.5 % respectively) [115].

In the Study of Trandolapril/Verapamil SR And Insulin Resistance (STAR) [116], a total of 240 hypertensive patients with impaired glucose tolerance were randomly assigned to the fixed-dose combinations of trandolapril/verapamil-SR or losartan/hydrochlorothiazide for 1 year long treatment period. This study examined the effects of these combinations on several parameters related to glycemic control, including glucose and insulin on 2-h of an oral glucose tolerance test (OGTT), HbA1c, IS, as well as incidence of new-onset diabetes. At 3 months of treatment significant differences in fasting glucose and IS and at study completion significant differences in 2-h OGTT-derived glucose and insulin levels and HbA1c were evident in favour of the trandolapril/verapamil-SR combination. Moreover, after 12 months of follow-up, the trandolapril/verapamil-SR combination was associated with a significantly lower risk of developing new-onset DM in comparison with the losartan/hydrochlorothiazide combination (11.0 % versus 26.6 % respectively, $P < 0.002$). This study advanced our knowledge in the field, showing for first time that even low doses of thiazide diuretics administered in combination with a "metabolic neutral" ARB can deteriorate glucose metabolism and elevate the risk of new-onset DM, providing opposite results to what was hypothesised until then [116].

Of major importance are also the results of the Diabetes Reduction Assessment with ramipril and rosiglitazone Medication (DREAM) trial, which had a 2×2 factorial design and randomly assigned 5,269 patients with impaired fasting glucose or impaired glucose tolerance to receive treatment with the ACEI ramipril (up to 15 mg daily) or placebo and rosiglitazone or placebo for a median follow-up period of 3 years [117]. The primary trial endpoint was the difference of these drugs on the incidence of new-onset DM or death, whichever occurred first. The occurrence of the primary outcome was similar between the ramipril (18.1 %) and the placebo groups (19.5 %) (HR 0.91; 95 % CI 0.81–1.03, $P = 0.15$). However, subjects receiving treatment with ramipril were more likely to present regression to normoglycemia than those receiving placebo (HR, 1.16; 95 % CI 1.07–1.27, $P = 0.001$), whereas plasma glucose levels 2 h after an OGTT were significantly lower in the ramipril group (135.1 vs 140.5 mg/dl, $P = 0.01$) [117]. In this context, the results of the DREAM trial suggested that treatment with ramipril for 3 years resulted in improvement of metabolic parameters and IS, despite the absence of any beneficial impact on the incidence of new-onset DM.

In addition to the above, a network meta-analysis that included 48 randomized groups from 22 clinical trials, involving 143,153 patients who did not have originally DM at randomization, aimed to provide a more conclusive answer to controversial issue of the effect of different classes of antihypertensive agents on incidence of new-onset DM [12]. Among 22 trials included in meta-analysis, 17 trials enrolled patients with hypertension, 3 trials enrolled patients at high cardiovascular risk and one trial recruited patients with HF. Using diuretic treatment as the standard of comparison, the odds ratios (OR) for the incidence of new-onset DM were 0.57 for ARBs (95 % CI 0.46–0.72, P < 0.001); 0.67 for ACEIs (95 % CI: 0.56–0.80, p < 0.001); 0.75 for CCBs (95 % CI: 0.62–0.90, P = 0.002); 0.77 for placebo 0.77 (95 % CI: 0.63–0.94, P = 0.009); and 0.90 for β-blockers (95 % CI: 0.75–1.09, P = 0.30). Thus, this meta-analysis clarified in a more straightforward way that the association of various antihypertensive drug classes with incidence of new-onset DM is lowest for ARBs and ACEIs, followed by CCBs and placebo, whereas β-blockers and diuretics are rather increasing DM incidence [12].

New-Onset DM and Cardiovascular Risk

All the evidence derived from large-scaled outcome trial presented above clearly suggest that thiazide diuretics and conventional β-blockers reduce IS, deteriorate glycemic control and heighten the risk of developing new-onset DM. A major aspect is whether and to what extent this antihypertensive therapy - induced elevation in incidence of new-onset DM affects cardiovascular morbidity and mortality of these patients. Verdecchia et al. attempted to explore this research question in a prospective cohort study including about 800 patients with never treated hypertension that were prospectively followed for a median period of 6 years. This study showed that patients who developed new-onset DM after the initiation of BP-lowering therapy carried a similar risk for experiencing subsequent cardiovascular events to that of patients who already had DM at study enrolment [118]. However, these findings contradict the results of the aforementioned SHEP trial [107], in which the thiazide diuretic-based antihypertensive regimen was associated with both better cardiovascular outcomes and elevated risk of developing new-onset DM relative to placebo. Further, in the ALLHAT trial, although chlorthalidone treatment was shown to be equally effective with lisinopril and amlodipine in reducing the risk of preventing cardiovascular events, incidence of new-onset DM was higher in the chlorthalidone than in the other two groups [100].

It has to be noted, however, that absence of association between thiazide diuretic-induced new-onset DM and increased risk of cardiovascular events in the above studies could be attributed to the short observation period after the development of DM [100, 107] that could not adequately capture the impact of this new DM on cardiovascular morbidity and mortality. Kostis et al. have attempted to clarify this issue in a study providing data on 14.3 years mean follow-up of the SHEP trial [119]. This study revealed that patients already being diabetic at randomization and patients who developed DM throughout the study in the placebo group had elevated risk of all-cause and cardiovascular mortality in contrast to patients who developed new-onset DM in the thiazide diuretic group, in whom diuretic-induced new-onset DM conferred no additional risk of all-cause and cardiovascular mortality [119]. On this basis, it has been proposed that adequate control of BP can possibly attenuate in the long term the expected elevation in cardiovascular risk from the development of new-onset DM related to the administration of antihypertensive treatment. This analysis, however, was substantially limited by the fact that the double-blind, randomized fashion of the trial ended in early 1991, after 4.3 years of follow-up, whereas the long-term data on the impact of antihypertensive treatment – related DM on cardiovascular outcomes were collected several years after the trial completion in an extended observational period, during which patients were receiving individualized BP-lowering treatment. Specifically-targeted research efforts are warranted in order to fully elucidate this intriguing issue. Until these arrive, the effects of diuretics and conventional β-blockers in elevating the incidence of DM should be taken seriously into account when physicians make their treatment decisions.

Conclusion

The choice of the appropriate antihypertensive treatment in patients with hypertension and HF should be influenced by the simultaneous presence of co-morbid conditions, such as CKD and DM. Major clinical trials evaluating the effects of RAAS blockers on hard renal outcomes have demonstrated that ACEIs and ARBs can slow the kidney injury progression in patients with diabetic or non-diabetic proteinuric CKD, and to delay the progression from micro- to macro-albuminuria in kidney diseases with predictable natural course (i.e. diabetic nephropathy). However, sub-analyses of major cardiovascular outcome trials suggest no specific benefit of RAAS blockade in normo-albuminuric patients with hypertension and preserved renal function and recent data suggest that dual ACEI/ARB inhibition produces more harm than good even in proteinuric CKD. In addition to the above, the effects of these agents on metabolic parameters and new-onset DM should be also taken into account when treatment regimens are planned. Use of thiazide diuretics and conventional β-blockers has been associated with deterioration in IS and elevated risk of developing new-onset DM, whereas newer vasodilating β-blockers, ACEIs, ARBs and CCBs were shown to have beneficial, or at least neutral, impact on metabolic profile. Since most patients with HF suffer from several co-morbidities, a careful consideration of the indications and contra-indications of the above commonly used agents remains a key to therapeutic success.

References

1. Yancy CW, Jessup M, Bozkurt B, et al. 2013 ACCF/AHA guideline for the management of heart failure: a report of the American College of Cardiology Foundation/American Heart Association Task Force on practice guidelines. Circulation. 2013;128:e240–319.
2. Go AS, Mozaffarian D, Roger VL, et al. Heart disease and stroke statistics – 2013 update: a report from the American Heart Association. Circulation. 2013;127:e6–245.
3. Curtis LH, Greiner MA, Hammill BG, et al. Early and long-term outcomes of heart failure in elderly persons, 2001–2005. Arch Intern Med. 2008;168:2481–8.
4. Curtis LH, Whellan DJ, Hammill BG, et al. Incidence and prevalence of heart failure in elderly persons, 1994–2003. Arch Intern Med. 2008;168:418–24.
5. Loehr LR, Rosamond WD, Chang PP, Folsom AR, Chambless LE. Heart failure incidence and survival (from the Atherosclerosis Risk in Communities study). Am J Cardiol. 2008;101:1016–22.
6. Roger VL, Weston SA, Redfield MM, et al. Trends in heart failure incidence and survival in a community-based population. JAMA. 2004;292:344–50.
7. Mancia G, Fagard R, Narkiewicz K, et al. 2013 ESH/ESC Guidelines for the management of arterial hypertension: the Task Force for the management of arterial hypertension of the European Society of Hypertension (ESH) and of the European Society of Cardiology (ESC). J Hypertens. 2013;31:1281–357.
8. Kidney Disease Outcomes Quality Initiative (K/DOQI). K/DOQI clinical practice guidelines on hypertension and antihypertensive agents in chronic kidney disease. Am J Kidney Dis. 2004;43:1–290.
9. Sarafidis PA, Ruilope LM. Aggressive blood pressure reduction and renin-angiotensin system blockade in chronic kidney disease: time for re-evaluation? Kidney Int. 2014;85(3):536–46.
10. Fried LF, Emanuele N, Zhang JH, et al. Combined angiotensin inhibition for the treatment of diabetic nephropathy. N Engl J Med. 2013;369:1892–903.

108   P.A. Sarafidis et al.

11. Parving HH, Brenner BM, McMurray JJ, et al. Cardiorenal end points in a trial of aliskiren for type 2 diabetes. N Engl J Med. 2012;367:2204–13.

12. Elliott WJ, Meyer PM. Incident diabetes in clinical trials of antihypertensive drugs: a network meta-analysis. Lancet. 2007;369:201–7.

13. Sarafidis PA, Bakris GL. Metabolic effects of beta-blockers: importance of dissociating newer from conventional agents. J Hypertens. 2007;25:249–52.

14. Sarafidis PA, McFarlane SI, Bakris GL. Antihypertensive agents, insulin sensitivity, and new-onset diabetes. Curr Diab Rep. 2007;7:191–9.

15. Lewis EJ, Hunsicker LG, Bain RP, Rohde RD. The effect of angiotensin-converting-enzyme inhibition on diabetic nephropathy. The Collaborative Study Group. N Engl J Med. 1993;329:1456–62.

16. Brenner BM, Cooper ME, de Zeeuw D, et al. Effects of losartan on renal and cardiovascular outcomes in patients with type 2 diabetes and nephropathy. N Engl J Med. 2001;345:861–9.

17. Lewis EJ, Hunsicker LG, Clarke WR, et al. Renoprotective effect of the angiotensin-receptor antagonist irbesartan in patients with nephropathy due to type 2 diabetes. N Engl J Med. 2001;345:851–60.

18. Strippoli GF, Craig M, Deeks JJ, Schena FP, Craig JC. Effects of angiotensin converting enzyme inhibitors and angiotensin II receptor antagonists on mortality and renal outcomes in diabetic nephropathy: systematic review. BMJ. 2004;329:828–38.

19. Sarafidis PA, Stafylas PC, Kanaki AI, Lasaridis AN. Effects of renin-angiotensin system blockers on renal outcomes and all-cause mortality in patients with diabetic nephropathy: an updated meta-analysis. Am J Hypertens. 2008;21:922–9.

20. De Zeeuw D, Remuzzi G, Parving HH, et al. Proteinuria, a target for renoprotection in patients with type 2 diabetic nephropathy: lessons from RENAAL. Kidney Int. 2004;65:2309–20.

21. Atkins RC, Briganti EM, Lewis JB, et al. Proteinuria reduction and progression to renal failure in patients with type 2 diabetes mellitus and overt nephropathy. Am J Kidney Dis. 2005;45:281–7.

22. The GISEN Group (Gruppo Italiano di Studi Epidemiologici in Nefrologia). Randomised placebo-controlled trial of effect of ramipril on decline in glomerular filtration rate and risk of

terminal renal failure in proteinuric, non-diabetic nephropathy. Lancet. 1997;349:1857–63.

23. Wright Jr JT, Bakris G, Greene T, et al. Effect of blood pressure lowering and antihypertensive drug class on progression of hypertensive kidney disease: results from the AASK trial. JAMA. 2002;288:2421–31.

24. Hou FF, Zhang X, Zhang GH, et al. Efficacy and safety of benazepril for advanced chronic renal insufficiency. N Engl J Med. 2006;354:131–40.

25. Jafar TH, Schmid CH, Landa M, et al. Angiotensin-converting enzyme inhibitors and progression of nondiabetic renal disease. A meta-analysis of patient-level data. Ann Intern Med. 2001;135:73–87.

26. Lea J, Greene T, Hebert L, et al. The relationship between magnitude of proteinuria reduction and risk of end-stage renal disease: results of the African American study of kidney disease and hypertension. Arch Intern Med. 2005;165:947–53.

27. Maschio G, Alberti D, Janin G, et al. Effect of the angiotensin-converting-enzyme inhibitor benazepril on the progression of chronic renal insufficiency. The Angiotensin-Converting-Enzyme Inhibition in Progressive Renal Insufficiency Study Group. N Engl J Med. 1996;334:939–45.

28. Jafar TH, Stark PC, Schmid CH, et al. Progression of chronic kidney disease: the role of blood pressure control, proteinuria, and angiotensin-converting enzyme inhibition: a patient-level meta-analysis. Ann Intern Med. 2003;139:244–52.

29. Ibsen H, Olsen MH, Wachtell K, et al. Reduction in albuminuria translates to reduction in cardiovascular events in hypertensive patients: losartan intervention for endpoint reduction in hypertension study. Hypertension. 2005;45:198–202.

30. Barnett AH, Bain SC, Bouter P, et al. Angiotensin-receptor blockade versus converting-enzyme inhibition in type 2 diabetes and nephropathy. N Engl J Med. 2004;351:1952–61.

31. Mangrum AJ, Bakris GL. Angiotensin-converting enzyme inhibitors and angiotensin receptor blockers in chronic renal disease: safety issues. Semin Nephrol. 2004;24:168–75.

32. Stafilas PC, Sarafidis PA, Lasaridis AN, Aletras VH, Niakas DA. An economic evaluation of the 2003 European Society of Hypertension-European Society of Cardiology guidelines for the management of mild-to-moderate hypertension in Greece. Am J Hypertens. 2005;18:1233–40.

33. Coresh J, Byrd-Holt D, Astor BC, et al. Chronic kidney disease awareness, prevalence, and trends among U.S. adults, 1999 to 2000. J Am Soc Nephrol. 2005;16:180–8.

34. O'Hare AM, Kaufman JS, Covinsky KE, Landefeld CS, McFarland LV, Larson EB. Current guidelines for using angiotensin-converting enzyme inhibitors and angiotensin II-receptor antagonists in chronic kidney disease: is the evidence base relevant to older adults? Ann Intern Med. 2009;150:717–24.

35. Casas JP, Chua W, Loukogeorgakis S, et al. Effect of inhibitors of the renin-angiotensin system and other antihypertensive drugs on renal outcomes: systematic review and meta-analysis. Lancet. 2005;366:2026–33.

36. de Zeeuw D, Lewis EJ, Remuzzi G, Brenner BM, Cooper ME. Renoprotective effects of renin-angiotensin-system inhibitors. Lancet. 2006;367:899–900.

37. Mann JF, McClellan WM, Kunz R, Ritz E. Progression of renal disease – can we forget about inhibition of the renin-angiotensin system? Nephrol Dial Transplant. 2006;21:2348–51.

38. Sarafidis PA, Khosla N, Bakris GL. Antihypertensive therapy in the presence of proteinuria. Am J Kidney Dis. 2007;49:12–26.

39. Rahman M, Pressel S, Davis BR, et al. Renal outcomes in high-risk hypertensive patients treated with an angiotensin-converting enzyme inhibitor or a calcium channel blocker vs a diuretic: a report from the Antihypertensive and Lipid-Lowering Treatment to Prevent Heart Attack Trial (ALLHAT). Arch Intern Med. 2005;165:936–46.

40. Estacio RO, Jeffers BW, Gifford N, Schrier RW. Effect of blood pressure control on diabetic microvascular complications in patients with hypertension and type 2 diabetes. Diabetes Care. 2000;23 Suppl 2:B54–64.

41. Bakris GL, Sarafidis PA, Weir MR, et al. Renal outcomes with different fixed-dose combination therapies in patients with hypertension at high risk for cardiovascular events (ACCOMPLISH): a prespecified secondary analysis of a randomised controlled trial. Lancet. 2010;375:1173–81.

42. Rossing K, Schjoedt KJ, Jensen BR, Boomsma F, Parving HH. Enhanced renoprotective effects of ultrahigh doses of irbesartan in patients with type 2 diabetes and microalbuminuria. Kidney Int. 2005;68:1190–8.

43. Schmieder RE, Klingbeil AU, Fleischmann EH, Veelken R, Delles C. Additional antiproteinuric effect of ultrahigh dose

candesartan: a double-blind, randomized, prospective study. J Am Soc Nephrol. 2005;16:3038–45.

44. Hollenberg NK, Parving HH, Viberti G, et al. Albuminuria response to very high-dose valsartan in type 2 diabetes mellitus. J Hypertens. 2007;25:1921–6.

45. Schjoedt KJ, Astrup AS, Persson F, et al. Optimal dose of lisinopril for renoprotection in type 1 diabetic patients with diabetic nephropathy: a randomised crossover trial. Diabetologia. 2009;52:46–9.

46. Mogensen CE, Neldam S, Tikkanen I, et al. Randomised controlled trial of dual blockade of renin-angiotensin system in patients with hypertension, microalbuminuria, and non-insulin dependent diabetes: the candesartan and lisinopril microalbuminuria (CALM) study. BMJ. 2000;321:1440–4.

47. Rossing K, Christensen PK, Jensen BR, Parving HH. Dual blockade of the renin-angiotensin system in diabetic nephropathy: a randomized double-blind crossover study. Diabetes Care. 2002;25:95–100.

48. Nakao N, Yoshimura A, Morita H, Takada M, Kayano T, Ideura T. Combination treatment of angiotensin-II receptor blocker and angiotensin-converting-enzyme inhibitor in non-diabetic renal disease (COOPERATE): a randomised controlled trial. Lancet. 2003;361:117–24.

49. Retraction – combination treatment of angiotensin-II receptor blocker and angiotensin-converting-enzyme inhibitor in non-diabetic renal disease (COOPERATE): a randomised controlled trial. Lancet. 2009;374:1226.

50. Mann JF, Schmieder RE, McQueen M, et al. Renal outcomes with telmisartan, ramipril, or both, in people at high vascular risk (the ONTARGET study): a multicentre, randomised, double-blind, controlled trial. Lancet. 2008;372:547–53.

51. Sarafidis PA, Bakris GL. Renin-angiotensin blockade and kidney disease. Lancet. 2008;372:511–2.

52. Ruilope LM, Segura J, Zamorano JL. New clinical concepts after the ONTARGET trial. Expert Rev Cardiovasc Ther. 2011;9:685–9.

53. Parving HH, Persson F, Lewis JB, Lewis EJ, Hollenberg NK. Aliskiren combined with losartan in type 2 diabetes and nephropathy. N Engl J Med. 2008;358:2433–46.

54. Persson F, Lewis JB, Lewis EJ, Rossing P, Hollenberg NK, Parving HH. Aliskiren in combination with losartan reduces albuminuria independent of baseline blood pressure in patients

with type 2 diabetes and nephropathy. Clin J Am Soc Nephrol. 2011;6:1025–31.

55. Novartis announces termination of ALTITUDE study with Rasilez®/Tekturna® in high-risk patients with diabetes and renal impairment. 4-1-2012. http://www.novartis.com/downloads/newsroom/rasilez-tekturna information-center/20111220-rasilez-tekturna.pdf. Accessed 4 January 2012.

56. Sarafidis PA, Bakris GL. Addition of renin-inhibitor in patients with chronic kidney disease: is it conclusively non-indicated? J Renin Angiotensin Aldosterone Syst. 2014;15(1):97–8.

57. Hollenberg NK. Aldosterone in the development and progression of renal injury. Kidney Int. 2004;66:1–9.

58. Bakris GL, Siomos M, Richardson D, et al. ACE inhibition or angiotensin receptor blockade: impact on potassium in renal failure. VAL-K Study Group. Kidney Int. 2000;58:2084–92.

59. Chrysostomou A, Pedagogos E, MacGregor L, Becker G. Aldosterone receptor antagonist spironolactone in patients who have persistent proteinuria and are on long-term angiotensin-converting enzyme inhibitor therapy, with or without an angiotensin II receptor blocker. Clin J Am Soc Nephrol. 2006;1:256–62.

60. Rossing K, Schjoedt KJ, Smidt UM, Boomsma F, Parving HH. Beneficial effects of adding spironolactone to recommended antihypertensive treatment in diabetic nephropathy: a randomized, double-masked, cross-over study. Diabetes Care. 2005;28:2106–12.

61. Schjoedt KJ, Rossing K, Juhl TR, et al. Beneficial impact of spironolactone in diabetic nephropathy. Kidney Int. 2005;68:2829–36.

62. Schjoedt KJ, Rossing K, Juhl TR, et al. Beneficial impact of spironolactone on nephrotic range albuminuria in diabetic nephropathy. Kidney Int. 2006;70:536–42.

63. Pitt B, Reichek N, Willenbrock R, et al. Effects of eplerenone, enalapril, and eplerenone/enalapril in patients with essential hypertension and left ventricular hypertrophy: the 4E-left ventricular hypertrophy study. Circulation. 2003;108:1831–8.

64. Mehdi UF, Adams-Huet B, Raskin P, Vega GL, Toto RD. Addition of angiotensin receptor blockade or mineralocorticoid antagonism to maximal angiotensin-converting enzyme inhibition in diabetic nephropathy. J Am Soc Nephrol. 2009;20:2641–50.

65. Sarafidis PA, Blacklock R, Wood E, et al. Prevalence and factors associated with hyperkalemia in predialysis patients followed in a low-clearance clinic. Clin J Am Soc Nephrol. 2012;7:1234–41.
66. Juurlink DN, Mamdani MM, Lee DS, et al. Rates of hyperkalemia after publication of the Randomized Aldactone Evaluation Study. N Engl J Med. 2004;351:543–51.
67. Pitt B, Zannad F, Remme WJ, et al. The effect of spironolactone on morbidity and mortality in patients with severe heart failure. Randomized Aldactone Evaluation Study Investigators. N Engl J Med. 1999;341:709–17.
68. Lind L, Berne C, Pollare T, Lithell H. Metabolic effects of anti-hypertensive treatment with nifedipine or furosemide: a double-blind, cross-over study. J Hum Hypertens. 1995;9:137–41.
69. Prince MJ, Stuart CA, Padia M, Bandi Z, Holland OB. Metabolic effects of hydrochlorothiazide and enalapril during treatment of the hypertensive diabetic patient. Enalapril for hypertensive diabetics. Arch Intern Med. 1988;148:2363–8.
70. Harper R, Ennis CN, Sheridan B, Atkinson AB, Johnston GD, Bell PM. Effects of low dose versus conventional dose thiazide diuretic on insulin action in essential hypertension. BMJ. 1994;309:226–30.
71. Harper R, Ennis CN, Heaney AP, et al. A comparison of the effects of low- and conventional-dose thiazide diuretic on insulin action in hypertensive patients with NIDDM. Diabetologia. 1995;38:853–9.
72. Hunter SJ, Harper R, Ennis CN, et al. Effects of combination therapy with an angiotensin converting enzyme inhibitor and thiazide diuretic on insulin action in essential hypertension. J Hypertens. 1998;16:103–9.
73. Hunter SJ, Wiggam MI, Ennis CN, et al. Comparison of effects of captopril used either alone or in combination with a thiazide diuretic on insulin action in hypertensive Type 2 diabetic patients: a double-blind crossover study. Diabet Med. 1999;16:482–7.
74. Sarafidis PA, Bakris GL. Do the metabolic effects of beta blockers make them leading or supporting antihypertensive agents in the treatment of hypertension? J Clin Hypertens (Greenwich). 2006;8:351–6.
75. Haenni A, Lithell H. Treatment with a beta-blocker with beta 2-agonism improves glucose and lipid metabolism in essential hypertension. Metabolism. 1994;43:455–61.

76. Jacob S, Rett K, Wicklmayr M, Agrawal B, Augustin HJ, Dietze GJ. Differential effect of chronic treatment with two beta-blocking agents on insulin sensitivity: the carvedilol-metoprolol study. J Hypertens. 1996;14:489–94.

77. Bakris GL, Fonseca V, Katholi RE, et al. Metabolic effects of carvedilol vs metoprolol in patients with type 2 diabetes mellitus and hypertension: a randomized controlled trial. JAMA. 2004;292:2227–36.

78. Giugliano D, Acampora R, Marfella R, et al. Metabolic and cardiovascular effects of carvedilol and atenolol in non-insulin-dependent diabetes mellitus and hypertension. A randomized, controlled trial. Ann Intern Med. 1997;126:955–9.

79. Poirier L, Cleroux J, Nadeau A, Lacourciere Y. Effects of nebivolol and atenolol on insulin sensitivity and haemodynamics in hypertensive patients. J Hypertens. 2001;19:1429–35.

80. Mason RP, Kalinowski L, Jacob RF, Jacoby AM, Malinski T. Nebivolol reduces nitroxidative stress and restores nitric oxide bioavailability in endothelium of black Americans. Circulation. 2005;112:3795–801.

81. Fogari R, Zoppi A, Lazzari P, et al. Comparative effects of nebivolol and atenolol on blood pressure and insulin sensitivity in hypertensive subjects with type II diabetes. J Hum Hypertens. 1997;11:753–7.

82. Kaiser T, Heise T, Nosek L, Eckers U, Sawicki PT. Influence of nebivolol and enalapril on metabolic parameters and arterial stiffness in hypertensive type 2 diabetic patients. J Hypertens. 2006;24:1397–403.

83. Ayers K, Byrne LM, DeMatteo A, Brown NJ. Differential effects of nebivolol and metoprolol on insulin sensitivity and plasminogen activator inhibitor in the metabolic syndrome. Hypertension. 2012;59:893–8.

84. Jauch KW, Hartl W, Guenther B, Wicklmayr M, Rett K, Dietze G. Captopril enhances insulin responsiveness of forearm muscle tissue in non-insulin-dependent diabetes mellitus. Eur J Clin Invest. 1987;17:448–54.

85. Suzuki M, Ikebuchi M, Yokota C, Shinozaki K, Harano Y. Normalization of insulin resistance in non-obese essential hypertension by cilazapril treatment. Clin Exp Hypertens. 1995;17:1257–68.

86. Zebekakis P, Kopras A, Lasaridis AN, et al. A comparative study of the effects of amlodipine and fosinopril on blood pres-

sure and insulin sensitivity in hypertensive patients. J Hypertens. 2003;21:S71.

87. Andersson PE, Lithell H. Metabolic effects of doxazosin and enalapril in hypertriglyceridemic, hypertensive men. Relationship to changes in skeletal muscle blood flow. Am J Hypertens. 1996;9:323–33.

88. Lender D, Arauz-Pacheco C, Breen L, Mora-Mora P, Ramirez LC, Raskin P. A double blind comparison of the effects of amlodipine and enalapril on insulin sensitivity in hypertensive patients. Am J Hypertens. 1999;12:298–303.

89. Kurtz TW. New treatment strategies for patients with hypertension and insulin resistance. Am J Med. 2006;119:S24–30.

90. Benson SC, Pershadsingh HA, Ho CI, et al. Identification of telmisartan as a unique angiotensin II receptor antagonist with selective PPARgamma-modulating activity. Hypertension. 2004;43:993–1002.

91. Sarafidis PA, Nilsson PM. The effects of thiazolidinediones on blood pressure levels – a systematic review. Blood Press. 2006;15:135–50.

92. Vitale C, Mercuro G, Castiglioni C, et al. Metabolic effect of telmisartan and losartan in hypertensive patients with metabolic syndrome. Cardiovasc Diabetol. 2005;4:6.

93. Sarafidis PA, Lasaridis AN, Hatzistavri L, Zebekakis P, Tziolas I. The effect of telmisartan and lercanidipine on blood pressure and insulin resistance in hypertensive patients. Rev Clin Pharmacol Pharmacokin (Int Ed). 2004;18:60–6.

94. Benndorf RA, Rudolph T, Appel D, et al. Telmisartan improves insulin sensitivity in nondiabetic patients with essential hypertension. Metabolism. 2006;55:1159–64.

95. Nagel JM, Tietz AB, Goke B, Parhofer KG. The effect of telmisartan on glucose and lipid metabolism in nondiabetic, insulin-resistant subjects. Metabolism. 2006;55:1149–54.

96. Grassi G, Seravalle G, Dell'Oro R, et al. Comparative effects of candesartan and hydrochlorothiazide on blood pressure, insulin sensitivity, and sympathetic drive in obese hypertensive individuals: results of the CROSS study. J Hypertens. 2003;21:1761–9.

97. Hansson L, Lindholm LH, Niskanen L, et al. Effect of angiotensin-converting-enzyme inhibition compared with conventional therapy on cardiovascular morbidity and mortality in hypertension: the Captopril Prevention Project (CAPPP) randomised trial. Lancet. 1999;353:611–6.

98. Brown MJ, Palmer CR, Castaigne A, et al. Morbidity and mortality in patients randomised to double-blind treatment with a long-acting calcium-channel blocker or diuretic in the International Nifedipine GITS study: Intervention as a Goal in Hypertension Treatment (INSIGHT). Lancet. 2000;356:366–72.

99. Dahlof B, Devereux RB, Kjeldsen SE, et al. Cardiovascular morbidity and mortality in the Losartan Intervention For Endpoint reduction in hypertension study (LIFE): a randomised trial against atenolol. Lancet. 2002;359:995–1003.

100. ALLHAT Officers and Coordinators for the ALLHAT Collaborative Research Group. Major outcomes in high-risk hypertensive patients randomized to angiotensin-converting enzyme inhibitor or calcium channel blocker vs diuretic: The Antihypertensive and Lipid-Lowering Treatment to Prevent Heart Attack Trial (ALLHAT). JAMA. 2002;288:2981–97.

101. Wing LM, Reid CM, Ryan P, et al. A comparison of outcomes with angiotensin-converting – enzyme inhibitors and diuretics for hypertension in the elderly. N Engl J Med. 2003; 348:583–92.

102. Reid CM, Johnston CI, Ryan P, WilLson K, Wing LM. Diabetes and cardiovascular outcomes in elderly subjects treated with ACE-inhibitors or diuretics: findings from the 2nd Australian National Blood Pressure Study. Am J Hypertens. 2003;16:11A.

103. Pepine CJ, Handberg EM, Cooper-DeHoff RM, et al. A calcium antagonist vs a non-calcium antagonist hypertension treatment strategy for patients with coronary artery disease. The International Verapamil-Trandolapril Study (INVEST): a randomized controlled trial. JAMA. 2003;290:2805–16.

104. Dahlof B, Sever PS, Poulter NR, et al. Prevention of cardiovascular events with an antihypertensive regimen of amlodipine adding perindopril as required versus atenolol adding bendroflumethiazide as required, in the Anglo-Scandinavian Cardiac Outcomes Trial-Blood Pressure Lowering Arm (ASCOT-BPLA): a multicentre randomised controlled trial. Lancet. 2005;366:895–906.

105. Yusuf S, Sleight P, Pogue J, Bosch J, Davies R, Dagenais G. Effects of an angiotensin-converting-enzyme inhibitor, ramipril, on cardiovascular events in high-risk patients. The Heart Outcomes Prevention Evaluation Study Investigators. N Engl J Med. 2000;342:145–53.

106. Pfeffer MA, Swedberg K, Granger CB, et al. Effects of candesartan on mortality and morbidity in patients with chronic heart failure: the CHARM-Overall programme. Lancet. 2003; 362:759–66.

107. SHEP Cooperative Research Group. Prevention of stroke by antihypertensive drug treatment in older persons with isolated systolic hypertension. Final results of the Systolic Hypertension in the Elderly Program (SHEP). JAMA. 1991;265:3255–64.

108. Padwal R, Laupacis A. Antihypertensive therapy and incidence of type 2 diabetes: a systematic review. Diabetes Care. 2004;27:247–55.

109. Hansson L, Lindholm LH, Ekbom T, et al. Randomised trial of old and new antihypertensive drugs in elderly patients: cardiovascular mortality and morbidity the Swedish Trial in Old Patients with Hypertension-2 study. Lancet. 1999;354:1751–6.

110. Hansson L, Hedner T, Lund-Johansen P, et al. Randomised trial of effects of calcium antagonists compared with diuretics and beta-blockers on cardiovascular morbidity and mortality in hypertension: the Nordic Diltiazem (NORDIL) study. Lancet. 2000;356:359–65.

111. Lithell H, Hansson L, Skoog I, et al. The Study on Cognition and Prognosis in the Elderly (SCOPE): principal results of a randomized double-blind intervention trial. J Hypertens. 2003;21:875–86.

112. Wilhelmsen L, Berglund G, Elmfeldt D, et al. Beta-blockers versus diuretics in hypertensive men: main results from the HAPPHY trial. J Hypertens. 1987;5:561–72.

113. Julius S, Kjeldsen SE, Weber M, et al. Outcomes in hypertensive patients at high cardiovascular risk treated with regimens based on valsartan or amlodipine: the VALUE randomised trial. Lancet. 2004;363:2022–31.

114. Kjeldsen SE, Julius S, Mancia G, et al. Effects of valsartan compared to amlodipine on preventing type 2 diabetes in high-risk hypertensive patients: the VALUE trial. J Hypertens. 2006;24:1405–12.

115. Lindholm LH, Persson M, Alaupovic P, Carlberg B, Svensson A, Samuelsson O. Metabolic outcome during 1 year in newly detected hypertensives: results of the Antihypertensive Treatment and Lipid Profile in a North of Sweden Efficacy Evaluation (ALPINE study). J Hypertens. 2003;21:1563–74.

116. Bakris G, Molitch M, Hewkin A, et al. Differences in glucose tolerance between fixed-dose antihypertensive drug combinations in people with metabolic syndrome. Diabetes Care. 2006;29:2592–7.
117. Bosch J, Yusuf S, Gerstein HC, et al. Effect of ramipril on the incidence of diabetes. N Engl J Med. 2006;355:1551–62.
118. Verdecchia P, Reboldi G, Angeli F, et al. Adverse prognostic significance of new diabetes in treated hypertensive subjects. Hypertension. 2004;43:963–9.
119. Kostis JB, Wilson AC, Freudenberger RS, Cosgrove NM, Pressel SL, Davis BR. Long-term effect of diuretic-based therapy on fatal outcomes in subjects with isolated systolic hypertension with and without diabetes. Am J Cardiol. 2005;95:29–35.

Chapter 4
Target Organ Damage and RAAS Blockade

Ilaria Spoletini, Cristiana Vitale, and Giuseppe M.C. Rosano

Introduction

The Renin – Angiotensin Aldosterone System (RAAS) plays a pivotal role in the regulation of blood pressure, plasma volume and sympathetic nervous system activity. By regulating body fluid volume perfusion, RAAS maintains systemic hemodynamic and hydromineral homeostasis. Thus, it protects the organs (i.e. heart, endothelium, brain, kidney) from

I. Spoletini, Ph.D.
Department of Medical Sciences, Centre for Clinical and Basic Research, IRCCS San Raffaele Pisana, via della Pisana, 235, Rome 00163, Italy

C. Vitale, M.D., Ph.D.
Department of Medical Sciences, Centre for Clinical and Basic Research, IRCCS San Raffaele Pisana, via della Pisana, 235, Rome 00163, Italy

Laboratory of Vascular Physiology, IRCCS San Raffaele, London, UK

G.M.C. Rosano, M.D., Ph.D., FESC, FACC (✉)
Department of Medical Sciences, Centre for Clinical and Basic Research, IRCCS San Raffaele Pisana, via della Pisana, 235, Rome 00163, Italy

Cardiovascular and Cell Science Institute, St Georges University, London, UK
e-mail: giuseppe.rosano@sanraffaele.it

© Springer International Publishing Switzerland 2015
P. Perrone Filardi (ed.), *ACEi and ARBS in Hypertension and Heart Failure*, Current Cardiovascular Therapy 5, DOI 10.1007/978-3-319-09788-6_4

chronic overexposure to elevated blood pressure, through a complex system of neuroendocrine interactions [60].

Conversely, chronic RAAS overactivation results in a cascade of proinflammatory, prothrombotic, and atherogenic events leading to target organ damage [60].

Inhibition of the RAAS is an effective therapeutic approach to prevent or limit target organ damage. RAAS may be inhibited at different levels: renin production and action, angiotensin I breakdown, angiotensin II action. Renin inhibitors (DRIs) block the conversion of angiotensinogen into angiotensin I and therefore inhibit the stimulatory effect of renin on the downstream activation of the system [45]. Angiotensin-converting enzyme inhibitors (ACEIs) block the conversion of angiotensin I into angiotensin II; angiotensin receptor blockers (ARBs) selectively inhibit angiotensin II from activating the angiotensin-specific receptor (angiotensin I). All of these interventions increase the upstream plasma renin levels and inhibit the negative feedback loop exerted by angiotensin II on renin production [3]. The most widely prescribed classes of drugs acting on the RAAS are ACEIs and ARBs, while the first DRI available for clinical use, aliskiren, was introduced in 2007.

Current evidence suggests that inhibition of the RAAS through ACEIs or ARBs allows blood pressure control and target-organ damage reduction [22]. However, translation of these benefits into reduction of mortality and morbidity has been proven only for ACE-I and is lacking for ARBs. Clinical trials have demonstrated that organ-protective effects may be obtained with both drugs in monotherapy, in patients with hypertension [1, 9, 24] and heart failure with left ventricular dysfunction [25, 55].

Due to the incomplete blockade with angiotensin I and renin accumulation [61] with ACEI or ARB monotherapy, determining subsequent 'escape' production of angiotensin II by non-ACE pathways, a better control of the RAAS system with the combination therapy (ARB + ACEI) has been hypothesised. This hypothesis does not take into account that for ACE-I with extensive tissue localisation like perindopril and ramipril the effect is not measurable by angiotensin I plasma level but rather by the tissue ACE enzyme activity.

It has been suggested that low doses of the two RAAS would have an enhanced effect, acting "synergistically" with a greater benefit for hypertension and nephroprotection [61]. Thus, combining ACEIs and ARBs has been thought to provide more extensive RAAS inhibition and greater antihypertensive efficacy and end-organ protection than use of either class alone [60]. This "more is better" hypothesis was proposed based on the findings from an animal study showing that dual therapy with enalapril and losartan had a greater effect on blood pressure and left ventricular weight/body weight ratio in a murine model of hypertension [33].

Nevertheless, the use of dual therapy ACEI + ARB on organ damage and other clinical outcomes in humans has been questioned, given conflicting results [11] and, above all, issues concerning safety.

Taking into account these issues, in this chapter we will examine the data on efficacy and safety of ACEIs and ARBs in arterial hypertension and heart failure, both in monotherapy or in combination, to clarify which of these therapeutic approaches may be an efficacious and safe strategy in patients with target organ damage, i.e. left ventricular hypertrophy and subclinical kidney dysfunction.

RAAS Dysregulation and Target Organ Damage

Organ damage, such as kidney disease and left ventricular hypertrophy, may occur as a consequence of a dysregulation of the RAAS system. The exact pathophysiological mechanisms activated by RAAS leading to target organ damage have been extensively reviewed [6, 8, 19, 21, 43, 48, 58].

Briefly, angiotensin I receptors are involved in mediating vasoconstriction, sympathetic nervous system activation, and cardiovascular remodeling. Angiotensin II receptors are implicated in vasodilation, antiproliferative effects, and apoptosis [19]. Angiotensin I is converted to angiotensin II by the angiotensin-converting enzyme present in the endothelial cells of the lung, vascular endothelium, and in the cell membranes of kidneys, heart, and brain. This system is also present in a wide variety of organs (tissue RAAS), allowing, also in the absence of circulating angiotensin I, the local synthesis of angiotensin II and the development of its autocrine or paracrine effects.

RAAS overactivation may contribute to renal disease because its role in the regulation of fluid–electrolyte balance [12]. In the kidney, the RAAS modifies plasma volume and cellular proliferation. In particular, constriction of the efferent arteriole by angiotensin II increases glomerular filtration by raising glomerular capillary pressure. The RAAS also increases sodium and water reabsorption through direct actions on renal tubular function. Thus, without intervention, from initial subclinical endothelial damage a decline in lomerular filtration rate occurs, macroalbuminuria develops, and eventually end-stage renal disease emerges [43].

Furthermore, RAAS over-activation in arterial hypertension causes left ventricular hypertrophy [18] whose main causal mechanisms are: (a) the increase in blood pressure, which leads to increased left ventricular wall stress; (b) aldosterone release from the adrenals and (c) direct action of angiotensin II on the cardiomyocytes [8].

Increased RAAS activity leads to hypertension and congestive heart failure because of its direct effects on vascular endothelial and smooth muscle cells [19]. Further, RAAS dysregulation is associated with amplification of events that contribute to vascular disease, such as inflammation and plaque formation and rupture [12]. In arterial hypertension the remodeling of the small arteries is one of the first manifestations of target organ damage, preceding the development of left ventricular hypertrophy, carotid artery intima-media thickening, or microalbuminuria.

By interrupting this cascade of events, RAAS blockade has a protective effect on heart and kidney disease as well as on arterial wall damage, in particular improving endothelial protection [19]. Since organ damage is associated with a significant increase in cardiovascular morbidity and mortality, the treatment of hypertension and heart failure is therefore aimed not only to decrease blood pressure, but also to prevent or reverse target organ damage.

For these reasons, RAAS inhibition represents first-line treatment for hypertensive and diabetic target organ damage, as well as preventing the progression of cardiovascular disease and kidney disease [21, 37]. Reduction of cardiorenal risk is a priority in patients at higher risk for damage, such as those with chronic kidney disease or heart failure with left ventricular dysfunction [58].

Monotherapy with ACEIs

A wealth amount of data has been cumulated to support the effect of ACEIs on end-organ protection (Table 4.1). One of the first clinical trials evaluating this outcome is the Collaborative Study Group trial, showing the efficacy of captopril (25 mg three times daily) compared to placebo, in reducing a combined endpoint of death, dialysis, and transplantation, thus improving renal function, in patients with type 1 diabetic patients [27]. In patients with asymptomatic left ventricular dysfunction after myocardial infarction, the Survival and Ventricular Enlargement trial (SAVE) [38] demonstrated that long-term administration of captopril was associated with an improvement in survival and reduced morbidity and mortality due to major cardiovascular events. In particular, a significant relative reduction in overall mortality of 19 % was observed in patients with left ventricular dysfunction, when added to standard therapy.

Further, the Studies of Left Ventricular Dysfunction (SOLVD) trial [55] and the Cooperative North Scandinavian Enalapril Survival Study (CONSENSUS) [53] demonstrated the beneficial effect of enalapril in reducing the number of fatal and nonfatal cardiovascular events in patients with heart failure. The CONSENSUS II trial [51] showed no improvement in survival or reduction in the rate of recurrent myocardial infarction. However, it demonstrated that patients receiving enalapril were less likely to require a change in therapy for treatment of heart failure.

The Heart Outcomes Prevention Evaluation (HOPE) [63] in patients with high cardiovascular risk (vascular disease or diabetes plus 1 other cardiovascular risk factor),

TABLE 4.1 Clinical trials with ACEIs in hypertension or heart failure

Trial	Drug	Patients	Primary outcomes	Main conclusions
SOLVD The SOLVD Investigators [55]	Enalapril vs placebo	6,797 patients with ejection fractions ≤ 0.35	Death from any cause, hospitalizations for heart failure	Enalapril reduced the incidence of heart failure and the rate of related hospitalizations in patients with asymptomatic left ventricular dysfunction. There was also a trend toward fewer deaths due to cardiovascular causes among the patients who received enalapril
CONSENSUS II Swedberg et al. [51]	Enalapril vs placebo	6,090 patients with acute myocardial infarctions and blood pressure above 100/60 mmHg	Death due to any cause within 6 months	Enalapril therapy started within 24 h of the onset of acute myocardial infarction did not improve survival during the 180 days after infarction

Study	Treatment	Patients	Endpoints	Results
AIRE The AIRE Study Investigators [52]	Ramipril vs placebo	2,006 patients with heart failure after an acute myocardial infarction	All-cause mortality Risk for death, severe/resistant heart failure, myocardial infarction, stroke	Mortality from all causes was significantly lower for patients randomised to receive ramipril. Analysis of prespecified secondary outcomes revealed a risk reduction of 19 %
TRACE Kober et al. [25]	Trandolapril vs placebo	1,749 patients with left ventricular ejection fraction ≤ 0.35	All-cause mortality Cardiovascular death, heart failure, recurrent myocardial infarction	Long-term treatment with trandolapril in patients with reduced left ventricular function soon after myocardial infarction significantly reduced the risk of overall mortality, mortality from cardiovascular causes, sudden death, and the development of severe heart failure

(continued)

TABLE 4.1 (continued)

Trial	Drug	Patients	Primary outcomes	Main conclusions
SAVE Rutherford et al. [44]	Captopril vs placebo	2,231 patients after an acute myocardial infarction with asymptomatic left ventricular dysfunction	Composite of recurrent myocardial infarction, cardiac revascularization and hospitalization for unstable angina	Captopril reduced recurrence of myocardial infarction and the need for cardiac revascularization but had no influence on the rate of hospitalization with a discharge diagnosis of unstable angina
BENEDICT-B Ruggenenti et al. [42]	Verapamil/ trandolapril vs trandolapril	281 hypertensive type 2 diabetes patients with microalbuminuria	Persistent macroalbuminuria (albuminuria >200 µg/ min in two consecutive visits). Treatment targets were systolic blood pressure/ diastolic blood pressure less than 120/80 mmHg and HbA1C less than 7 %	Verapamil added on trandolapril did not improve renal or cardiovascular outcomes. Independent of verapamil, trandolapril normalized albuminuria in half of patients and this translated into significant cardioprotection

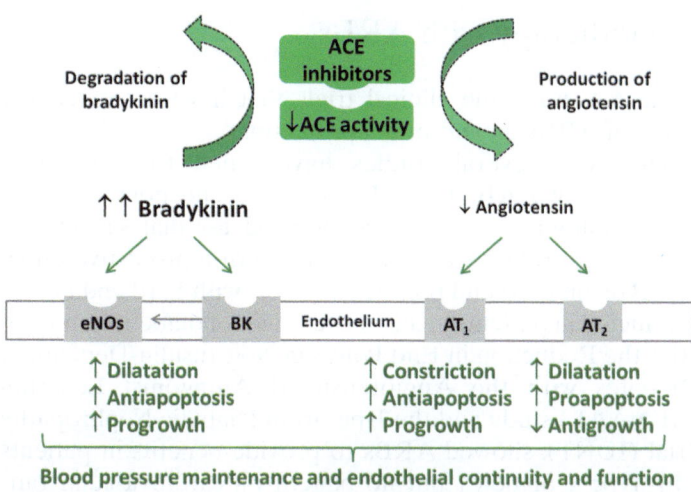

FIG. 4.1 Mechanisms of action of ACEIs (Adapted from Ferrari and Rosano [15])

showed that treatment with ramipril 10 mg/day reduced the risk of cardiovascular death, myocardial infarction and stroke, compared with placebo. In patients with coronary artery disease, the EURopean trial On reduction of cardiac events with Perindopril in stable coronary Artery disease (EUROPA) [16] found that perindopril 8 mg/day reduced the risk for the composite end point of cardiovascular death, myocardial infarction and cardiac arrest compared with placebo.

The efficacy of long-term ACEI monotherapy in reducing cardiovascular risk and protecting end-organ function and reducing cardiovascular events beyong blood pressure reduction is therefore well established, as recently reviewed [29]. Several other trials consistently indicated that ACE monotherapy improved cardiovascular outcomes in patients with hypertension or heart failure [25, 42, 52]. The mechanisms of action of ACE inhibition that may explain these results are shown in Fig. 4.1.

Monotherapy with ARBs

Table 4.2 shows the clinical trials that have evaluated the effect of ARBs on end-organ protection.

However, several studies have failed to show non-inferiority of ARBs to ACEIs on hard end points such as death, doubling of creatinine or need for dialysis, and no placebo-controlled study has ever shown a protective effect of ARBs on hard end points. Two trials with hard end points, conducted in patients in advanced stages of diabetic nephropathy, the Reduction in End Points in Non-Insulin-Dependent Diabetes with the Angiotensin II Antagonist Losartan (RENAAL) study and the Irbesartan Diabetic Nephropathy Trial (IDNT), showed ARBs to provide benefits in patients with type 2 diabetes, but no benefit on cardiovascular outcomes was statistically significant. Thus, ARBs do not reduce cardiovascular events.

Two other studies – the Irbesartan Microalbuminuria Study (IRMA)-2 [36] and the Microalbuminuria Reduction with Valsartan study (MARVAL) [59] – showed the efficacy of ARBs in reducing microalbuminuria, a surrogate endpoint associated with early-stage diabetic nephropathy. Similarly, the Telmisartan Randomised Assessment Study in ACE Intolerant Subjects with Cardiovascular Disease (TRANSCEND) trial [64] found the efficacy of telmisartan on the following surrogate end points: serum creatinine, estimated glomerular filtration rate and albuminuria. These data are therefore not sufficient to draw conclusions on the efficacy of ARBs in reducing diabetic nephropathy. Indeed, whether the effect of ARBs on surrogate end points translates into a prognostic benefit is unknown.

Further, there is evidence from the Valsartan Heart Failure Trial (Val-HeFT) [7] that valsartan had a significant effect in reducing the mortality rate when added to standard therapy with heart failure, but not in the subgroup of patients taking an ACEI or a beta-blocker. In elderly patients with heart failure, the Irbesartan in heart failure

TABLE 4.2 Clinical trials with ARBs in hypertension or heart failure

Trial	Drug	Patients	Primary outcomes	Main conclusions
TRANSCEND Yusuf et al. [64]	Telmisartan vs placebo	5,927 ACEI intolerant patients with coronary, peripheral or cerebrovascular disease or diabetes with end-organ damage; controlled blood pressure	Composite endpoint of cardiovascular death, non-fatal myocardial infarction, non-fatal stroke and hospitalization for congestive heart failure	In adults with vascular disease but without macroalbuminuria, the effects of telmisartan on major renal outcomes were similar to those of placebo
I-PRESERVE Massie et al. [31]	Irbesartan vs placebo	4,100 patients with chronic heart failure and relative preserved LV function	Composite outcome of death (all cause) and prespecified cardiovascular hospital admissions	Irbesartan did not improve the outcomes of patients with heart failure and a preserved left ventricular ejection fraction

(continued)

TABLE 4.2 (continued)

Trial	Drug	Patients	Primary outcomes	Main conclusions
SCOPE Lithell et al. [28]	Candesartan vs placebo	4,964 elderly patients	Composite outcome of cardiovascular death, non-fatal stroke and non-fatal myocardial infarction Secondary outcome measures included cardiovascular death, non-fatal and fatal stroke and myocardial infarction, cognitive function	A slightly more effective blood pressure reduction with candesartan was associated with a with a marked reduction in non-fatal stroke. Only a modest, statistically non-significant, reduction in major cardiovascular events was observed
LIFE Dahlof et al. [9]	Losartan vs atenolol	9,193 patients aged 55–80 years with essential hypertension and left ventricular hypertrophy	Composite of death, myocardial infarction and stroke	Losartan prevented more cardiovascular morbidity and death than atenolol for a similar reduction in blood pressure and was better tolerated

VALUE Julius et al. [24]	Valsartan vs amlodipine	15,245 patients with hypertension and high cardiovascular risk	Composite of cardiovascular death and cardiovascular events	The main outcome of cardiac disease did not differ between the treatment groups. Blood pressure was reduced by both treatments, but the effects of the amlodipine-based regimen were more pronounced, especially in the early period
CHARM-Alternative Granger et al. [20]	Candesartan vs placebo	2,028 patients with chronic heart failure, left ventricular dysfunction and ACEI intolerance	Composite of cardiovascular death and heart failure hospitalization	Candesartan was generally well tolerated and reduced cardiovascular mortality and morbidity

(continued)

TABLE 4.2 (continued)

Trial	Drug	Patients	Primary outcomes	Main conclusions
Val-HeFT Cohn et al. [7]	Valsartan vs placebo added to standard therapy for heart failure	5,010 patients with chronic heart failure	Combined endpoint of cardiovascular morbidity and mortality	Valsartan significantly reduced the combined end point and improved clinical signs and symptoms of heart failure, when added to prescribed therapy. However, when added to an ACEI or a beta-blocker the addition of valsartan had an adverse effect in terms mortality and morbidity
MOSES Schrader et al. [49]	Eprosartan vs nitrendipine	1,405 high-risk hypertensive patients with history of stroke	Composite of all-cause mortality, cardiovascular and cerebrovascular events	An early normotensive and comparable blood pressure was achieved. The combined end point was significantly lower in the eprosartan group

with Preserved systolic function (I-PRESERVE) trial [31] studied the effect of irbesartan 300 mg/die on a primary composite outcome of death from any cause or hospitalisation for a cardiovascular cause. Secondary outcomes included death from heart failure or hospitalisation for heart failure, death from any cause and from cardiovascular causes, and quality of life. No significant differences in the outcomes were found. However, a subsequent sub-analysis of the trial [26] showed differential results for gender. Women (n = 2,491) with heart failure with preserved ejection fraction were more likely to have chronic kidney disease and hypertension than men. Thus, given these results, it may be relevant to assess the sex differences in risk among patients with heart failure.

Other ARBs, such as eprosartan [49] and candesartan [28], have been evaluated in clinical trials. The Candesartan in Heart Failure-Assessment of Reduction in Mortality and Morbidity (CHARM) trial [40] compared the effects of candesartan and placebo added to existing antihypertensive therapy in patients with chronic heart failure and left ventricular ejection fraction <40 %, finding that candesartan significantly reduced cardiovascular deaths and hospital admissions for heart failure. CHARM-Alternative [20] further evaluated candesartan therapy compared with placebo in patients who were intolerant to ACEIs, showing its effectiveness in reducing the incidence of cardiovascular death or hospital admission for heart failure. However, in patients with symptomatic heart failure but preserved systolic function in CHARM-Preserved [62], candesartan treatment was not associated with significant benefit.

In conclusions, ARBs have been reported to have some beneficial effects only on surrogate end points associated with heart and kidney disease progression. There is evidence that ARBs may blunt progression of advanced diabetic nephropathy (see Fig. 4.2 for mechanisms of action), but their long-term renal effects in other patients are not clear.

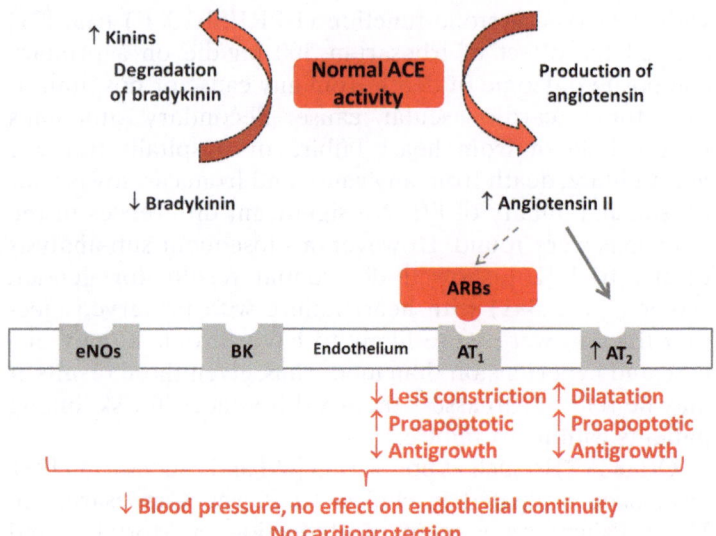

Fig. 4.2 Mechanisms of action of ARBs (Adapted from Ferrari and Rosano [15])

Dual Therapy

Clinical trials have investigated the efficacy of dual therapy (ACEI + ARB) on cardiovascular and renal outcomes [2, 32, 34, 39]. Five trials have evaluated the effects of combination therapy with an ACEI and an ARB compared with treatment with either agent alone (Table 4.3).

In 2003, the Combination Treatment of Angiotensin-II Receptor Blocker and Angiotensin-Converting-Enzyme Inhibitor in Non-Diabetic Renal Disease (COOPERATE) trial showed data apparently supporting the use of dual RAAS blockade, but the validity of these data was questioned, leading to its retraction [54].

The Avoiding Cardiovascular Events through Combination Therapy in Patients Living with Systolic Hypertension (ACCOMPLISH) trial [23] showed that the combination of benazepril plus amlodipine was more effective than benazepril

TABLE 4.3 Clinical trials combining ACEI+ARB and clinical trials comparing ACEIs and ARBs in hypertension or heart failure

Trial	Drug	Patients	Primary outcomes	Main conclusions
ONTARGET Yusuf et al. [64]	Telmisartan and ramipril both in monotherapy and combined	23,400 high risk patients with coronary, peripheral or cerebrovascular disease or diabetes with end-organ damage; controlled BP	Composite endpoint of cardiovascular death, non-fatal myocardial infarction, non-fatal stroke and hospitalization for congestive heart failure	In people at high vascular risk, the treatment effects on major renal outcomes were similar. Although combination therapy reduced proteinuria to a greater extent than monotherapy, overall it worsened major renal outcomes
ELITE Pitt et al. [41]	Losartan vs captopril	722 ACE-inhibitor naive patients aged ≥65 years with NYHA class II-IV heart failure and ejection fractions ≤40 %	Safety measure of renal dysfunction, composite of death and/or hospital admission for heart failure; and other efficacy measures	Treatment with losartan was associated with lower mortality than captopril. No difference in renal dysfunction was observed

(continued)

TABLE 4.3 (continued)

Trial	Drug	Patients	Primary outcomes	Main conclusions
CHARM-Added McMurray et al. [32]	Candesartan vs placebo added to ACE inhibitor	2,548 patients with heart failure and left ventricular ejection fraction ≤40 %	Composite of cardiovascular death and heart failure hospitalization	Candesartan reduced each of the components of the primary outcome significantly, as well as the total number of hospital admissions for heart failure. The benefits of candesartan were similar in all predefined subgroups, including patients receiving baseline beta blocker treatment
VALIANT Pfeffer et al. [39, 40]	Valsartan, captopril or both	14,703 patients with acute myocardial infarction and heart failure, left ventricular dysfunction or both	All-cause mortality	Valsartan was as effective as captopril in patients at high risk for cardiovascular events after myocardial infarction. Combining valsartan with captopril increased the rate of adverse events without improving survival

| CALM Mogensen et al. [34] | Candesartan plus lisinopril vs candesartan and lisinopril alone | 199 patients with hypertension, type II diabetes, microalbuminuria | Change in blood pressure and UA:Cr ratio | Candesartan was as effective as lisinopril in reducing blood pressure and microalbuminuria in hypertensive patients with type 2 diabetes |
| IMPROVE Bakris et al. [2] | Irbesartan ramipril or both | 405 patients with hypertension, microalbuminuria, high risk for cardiovascular events | Reduction in urinary albumin excretion | No differences between treatments for the endpoint. Although differences in blood pressure reductions were observed between the two treatments, these changes did not affect microalbuminuria. The incidence of adverse effects and treatment-related adverse effects was similar in both groups |

(continued)

TABLE 4.3 (continued)

Trial	Drug	Patients	Primary outcomes	Main conclusions
OPTIMAAL Dickstein et al. [10]	Losartan vs captopril	5,477 patients with acute myocardial infarction and heart failure or left ventricular dysfunction	All cause mortality Myocardial infarction – related death, cardiovascular death, stroke	No differences between treatments for any endpoints. Losartan was significantly better tolerated than captopril, with fewer patients discontinuing study medication
VA NEPHRON-D Fried et al. [17]	Losartan plus lisinopril or placebo	Patients with type 2 diabetes and urinary albumin-to-creatinine ratio of at least 300, and GFR 30.0–89.9 ml per minute per 1.73 m^2 of body-surface area	Change in the estimated GFR, end-stage renal disease or death The secondary renal end point was the first occurrence of a decline in the estimated GFR or end-stage renal disease Safety outcomes included mortality, hyperkalemia, and acute kidney injury	The study was discontinued due to safety concerns. Combination therapy increased the risk of hyperkalemia and acute kidney injury A trend toward a benefit from combination therapy with respect to the secondary end point decreased with time. There was no benefit with respect to mortality or cardiovascular events

alone in reducing cardiovascular events. There was a small difference in systolic blood pressure between the groups showing a slight benefit with benazcpril plus amlodipine.

Another study, the Ongoing Telmisartan Alone and in Combination with Ramipril Trial (ONTARGET) [30], investigated the renal effects of ramipril, telmisartan, and their combination in patients aged 55 years or older with established atherosclerotic vascular disease or with diabetes with end-organ damage. The combined therapy did not reduce the risk of renal and cardiovascular outcomes compared with the single use of either agent. Dual therapy, notably, significantly increased the risk of hypotension, syncope, renal dysfunction, and hyperkalemia, with a trend toward an increased risk of renal dysfunction requiring dialysis.

Also, the Veterans Affairs Nephropathy in Diabetes (VA NEPHRON-D) [17] studied the effects of lisinopril, losartan, and their combination in patients with type 2 diabetes. The primary endpoint was a decrease in glomerular filtration rate, end-stage renal disease, or death. The secondary endpoint was the first occurrence of a glomerular filtration rate decline or end-stage renal disease. Also this trial was discontinued due to safety concerns, i.e. the occurrence of hyperkalemic events and of acute kidney injury, with no differences for the endpoint outcomes.

Recently, the Progresión de Nefropatía Diabética (PRONEDI) study investigated the efficacy of lisinopril, irbesartan both in monotherapy or combined, in reducing the progression of type 2 diabetic nephropathy [13]. The study did not show a benefit of the dual therapy compared to monotherapy on the risk of progression of type 2 diabetic nephropathy. The number of adverse events including hyperkalemia was similar in all three groups. However, limitations of the study are that the sample size is small (n = 133) and the study is not double blind.

Taken all together, these studies consistently demonstrated that the combination of ACEI and ARB leads to higher risk of adverse events, i.e. increased risk of hypotension, hyperkalemia and renal failure, without improved efficacy.

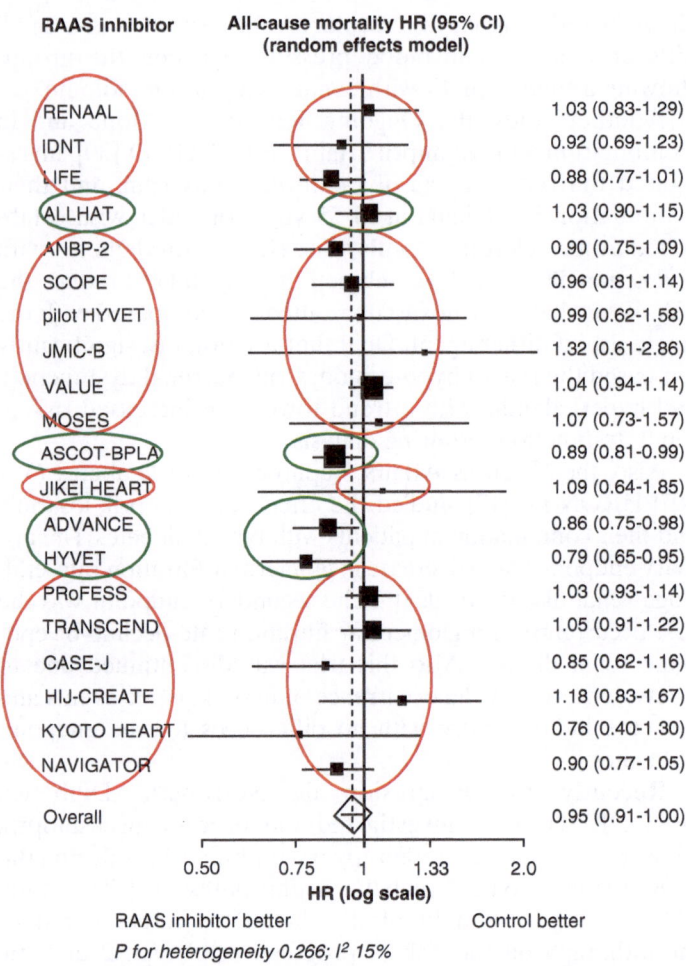

Fɪɢ. 4.3 "Findings from the meta-analyses on ARBs and ACEIs. Studies on ACEIs are circled in *green*, studies on ARBs are circled in *red* (Adapted from Ferrari and Rosano [15])

This conclusion has been also substantiated by several meta-analyses, that are shown in Fig. 4.3. Strong evidence shows that dual RAAS blockade does not offer additional benefit than monotherapy in reducing overall mortality, cardiovascular mortality or stroke, but increases the risks of hyperkalemia, hypotension, renal failure and treatment discontinuation due to adverse effects.

Comparison Between ACEIs and ARBs

In order to clarify whether monotherapy with an ACEI or with an ARB is preferable, the Telmisartan versus Ramipril in renal ENdothelial DYsfunction in type 2 diabetes (TRENDY) study [47] investigated the effect of telmisartan or ramipril in renal endothelial function in patients with diabetes and hypertension at high risk of cardiovascular and renal morbidity. The TRENDY is a stand-alone trial and part of the ongoing Programme of Research to Show Telmisartan End-Organ Protection (PROTECTION) Study Programme. Both treatments were associated with an increase in basal nitric oxide activity of the renal endothelium, which indicates an improvement from renal endothelial dysfunction [47]. ARBs and ACEIs (i.e. telmisartan and enalapril) were also found to be similarly effective in reducing long-term renal decline, as shown in the Diabetics Exposed to Telmisartan And enalaprIL (DETAIL) trial [5]. Other trials [10, 41] comparing the efficacy of an ACEI and an ARB are shown in Table 4.3.

However, several large meta-analyses have compared the effect of ACEIs and ARBs [4, 14, 46, 50, 56, 57]. In particular, while both classes of drugs reduce blood pressure, ACEIs are better than ARBs in coronary prevention and in the reduction of overall mortality and pneumonia. The consistent conclusion is that ACEIs prevent coronary events with reductions in cardiovascular morbidity and mortality endpoints, while ARBs are, at best, only effective for the prevention of stroke [15]. In conclusion, results from meta-analyses have clarified the superiority of ACEIs over ARBs in reducing cardiovascular mortality and the risk of organ damage. Renin inhibition should be solely limited to blood pressure reduction. There is now clear evidence that double blockade of the RAS is detrimental and must not be used in clinical practice. It is important to consider that, given the mortality benefit of ACE-inhibitors, a preferential first line use of ARBs poses important public health implications.

Conclusions

Considering data from meta-analyses and individual randomised trials, dual RAAS blockade is not advisable, being associated with increased risk of adverse events compared to monotherapy without significant benefit in patients. Patients with established cardio-renal disease may be at more risk of adverse effects when a second RAAS blocker is introduced [17, 35, 64]. Thus, as pointed out by EMA and current European Society of Cardiology-European Society of Hypertension 2013 guidelines for the management of arterial hypertension, combination therapy with ACEI + ARB should be discouraged and only limited to selected patient groups, e.g. chronic heart failure patients with persisting symptoms who cannot take mineralocorticoids. Dual RAAS blockade of ACEIs and ARBs is particularly contraindicated in patients with diabetes and severe renal impairment.

Taken all together, a large body of data show that both ARBs and ACEIs in monotherapy have an efficacy in blood pressure reduction and target organ damage [22], but there is more support for the use of ACEIs for the management of hypertension, heart failure and their consequence on organ damage. In particular, ARBs have failed to show superiority to ACEIs in reducing cardiovascular events and in some cases have raised concerns about the safety of long-term treatment with ARBs. These results indicate that the two classes of drugs should not be considered interchangeable [15] and ACEIs should be preferred to ARBs in patients with hypertension and heart failure to reduce cardiovascular events and target organ damage.

References

1. ALLHAT Officers and Coordinators for the ALLHAT Collaborative Research Group, The Antihypertensive and Lipid-Lowering Treatment to Prevent Heart Attack Trial. Major outcomes in high-risk hypertensive patients randomized to angiotensin-converting enzyme inhibitor or calcium channel blocker vs diuretic: The Antihypertensive and Lipid-Lowering Treatment to Prevent Heart Attack Trial (ALLHAT). JAMA. 2002;288:2981–97.

2. Bakris GL, Ruilope L, Locatelli F, et al. Treatment of microalbuminuria in hypertensive subjects with elevated cardiovascular risk: results of the IMPROVE trial. Kidney Int. 2007;72:879–85.

3. Balakumar P, Jagadeesh G. Cardiovascular and renal pathologic implications of prorenin, renin, and the (pro)renin receptor: promising young players from the old renin-angiotensin-aldosterone system. J Cardiovasc Pharmacol. 2010;56:570–9.

4. Bangalore S, Kumar S, Wetterslev J, et al. Angiotensin receptor blockers and risk of myocardial infarction: meta-analyses and trial sequential analyses of 147 020 patients from randomised trials. BMJ. 2011;342:d2234.

5. Barnett AH, Bain SC, Bouter P, et al. Angiotensin-receptor blockade versus converting-enzyme inhibition in type 2 diabetes and nephropathy. N Engl J Med. 2004;351:1952–61.

6. Bidani AK, Griffin KA, Epstein M. Hypertension and chronic kidney disease progression: why the suboptimal outcomes? Am J Med. 2012;125:1057–62.

7. Cohn JN, Tognoni G, Valsartan Heart Failure Trial I. A randomized trial of the angiotensin-receptor blocker valsartan in chronic heart failure. N Engl J Med. 2001;345:1667–75.

8. Cowan BR, Young AA. Left ventricular hypertrophy and renin-angiotensin system blockade. Curr Hypertens Rep. 2009; 11:167–72.

9. Dahlof B, Devereux RB, Kjeldsen SE, et al. Cardiovascular morbidity and mortality in the Losartan Intervention For Endpoint reduction in hypertension study (LIFE): a randomised trial against atenolol. Lancet. 2002;359:995–1003.

10. Dickstein K, Kjekshus J, OPTIMAAL Steering Committee of the OPTIMAAL Study Group. Effects of losartan and captopril on mortality and morbidity in high-risk patients after acute myocardial infarction: the OPTIMAAL randomised trial.

Optimal Trial in Myocardial Infarction with Angiotensin II Antagonist Losartan. Lancet. 2002;360:752–60.

11. Dusing R, Sellers F. ACE inhibitors, angiotensin receptor blockers and direct renin inhibitors in combination: a review of their role after the ONTARGET trial. Curr Med Res Opin. 2009; 25:2287–301.

12. Dzau VJ. Theodore Cooper Lecture: tissue angiotensin and pathobiology of vascular disease: a unifying hypothesis. Hypertension. 2001;37:1047–52.

13. Fernandez Juarez G, Luno J, Barrio V, et al. Effect of dual blockade of the renin-angiotensin system on the progression of type 2 diabetic nephropathy: a randomized trial. Am J Kidney Dis. 2013;61:211–8.

14. Ferrari R, Boersma E. The impact of ACE inhibition on all-cause and cardiovascular mortality in contemporary hypertension trials: a review. Expert Rev Cardiovasc Ther. 2013;11:705–17.

15. Ferrari R, Rosano GM. Not just numbers, but years of science: putting the ACE inhibitor-ARB meta-analyses into context. Int J Cardiol. 2013;166(2):286–8.

16. Fox KM. Efficacy of perindopril in reduction of cardiovascular events among patients with stable coronary artery disease: randomised, double-blind, placebo-controlled, multicentre trial (the EUROPA study). Lancet. 2003;362:782–8.

17. Fried LF, Emanuele N, Zhang JH, et al. Combined angiotensin inhibition for the treatment of diabetic nephropathy. N Engl J Med. 2013;369:1892–903.

18. Gosse P. Left ventricular hypertrophy – the problem and possible solutions. J Int Med Res. 2005;33 Suppl 1:3A–11.

19. Grandi AM, Maresca AM. Blockade of the renin-angiotensin-aldosterone system: effects on hypertensive target organ damage. Cardiovasc Hematol Agents Med Chem. 2006;4:219–28.

20. Granger CB, McMurray JJ, Yusuf S, et al. Effects of candesartan in patients with chronic heart failure and reduced left-ventricular systolic function intolerant to angiotensin-converting-enzyme inhibitors: the CHARM-Alternative trial. Lancet. 2003;362:772–6.

21. Hayashi T, Takai S, Yamashita C. Impact of the renin-angiotensin-aldosterone-system on cardiovascular and renal complications in diabetes mellitus. Curr Vasc Pharmacol. 2010;8:189–97.

22. Houston Miller N. Cardiovascular risk reduction with renin-angiotensin aldosterone system blockade. Nurs Res Pract. 2010;2010:101749.

23. Jamerson K, Bakris GL, Dahlof B, et al. Exceptional early blood pressure control rates: the ACCOMPLISH trial. Blood Press. 2007;16:80–6.

24. Julius S, Kjeldsen SE, Weber M, et al. Outcomes in hypertensive patients at high cardiovascular risk treated with regimens based on valsartan or amlodipine: the VALUE randomised trial. Lancet. 2004;363:2022–31.

25. Kober L, Torp-Pedersen C, Carlsen JE, et al. A clinical trial of the angiotensin-converting-enzyme inhibitor trandolapril in patients with left ventricular dysfunction after myocardial infarction. Trandolapril Cardiac Evaluation (TRACE) Study Group. N Engl J Med. 1995;333:1670–6.

26. Lam CS, Carson PE, Anand IS, et al. Sex differences in clinical characteristics and outcomes in elderly patients with heart failure and preserved ejection fraction: the Irbesartan in Heart Failure with Preserved Ejection Fraction (I-PRESERVE) trial. Circ Heart Fail. 2012;5:571–8.

27. Lewis EJ, Hunsicker LG, Bain RP, et al. The effect of angiotensin-converting-enzyme inhibition on diabetic nephropathy. The Collaborative Study Group. N Engl J Med. 1993;329:1456–62.

28. Lithell H, Hansson L, Skoog I, et al. The Study on Cognition and Prognosis in the Elderly (SCOPE): principal results of a randomized double-blind intervention trial. J Hypertens. 2003;21:875–86.

29. Luft FC. Perspective on combination RAS blocking therapy: Off-TARGET, Dis-CORD, MAP-to-nowhere, low ALTITUDE, and NEPHRON-D. Am J Nephrol. 2014;39:46–9.

30. Mann JF, Schmieder RE, McQueen M, et al. Renal outcomes with telmisartan, ramipril, or both, in people at high vascular risk (the ONTARGET study): a multicentre, randomised, double-blind, controlled trial. Lancet. 2008;372:547–53.

31. Massie BM, Carson PE, McMurray JJ, et al. Irbesartan in patients with heart failure and preserved ejection fraction. N Engl J Med. 2008;359:2456–67.

32. McMurray JJ, Ostergren J, Swedberg K, et al. Effects of candesartan in patients with chronic heart failure and reduced left-ventricular systolic function taking angiotensin-converting-enzyme inhibitors: the CHARM-Added trial. Lancet. 2003;362:767–71.

33. Menard J, Campbell DJ, Azizi M, et al. Synergistic effects of ACE inhibition and Ang II antagonism on blood pressure, cardiac weight, and renin in spontaneously hypertensive rats. Circulation. 1997;96:3072–8.

34. Mogensen CE, Neldam S, Tikkanen I, et al. Randomised controlled trial of dual blockade of renin-angiotensin system in patients with hypertension, microalbuminuria, and non-insulin dependent diabetes: the candesartan and lisinopril microalbuminuria (CALM) study. BMJ. 2000;321:1440–4.

35. Parving HH, Brenner BM, McMurray JJ, et al. Cardiorenal end points in a trial of aliskiren for type 2 diabetes. N Engl J Med. 2012;367:2204–13.

36. Parving HH, Lehnert H, Brochner-Mortensen J, et al. The effect of irbesartan on the development of diabetic nephropathy in patients with type 2 diabetes. N Engl J Med. 2001;345:870–8.

37. Pende A, Dallegri F. Renin-angiotensin antagonists: therapeutic effects beyond blood pressure control? Curr Pharm Des. 2012;18:1011–20.

38. Pfeffer MA, Braunwald E, Moye LA, et al. Effect of captopril on mortality and morbidity in patients with left ventricular dysfunction after myocardial infarction. Results of the survival and ventricular enlargement trial. The SAVE Investigators. N Engl J Med. 1992;327:669–77.

39. Pfeffer MA, McMurray JJ, Velazquez EJ, et al. Valsartan, captopril, or both in myocardial infarction complicated by heart failure, left ventricular dysfunction, or both. N Engl J Med. 2003;349:1893–906.

40. Pfeffer MA, Swedberg K, Granger CB, et al. Effects of candesartan on mortality and morbidity in patients with chronic heart failure: the CHARM-Overall programme. Lancet. 2003; 362:759–66.

41. Pitt B, Segal R, Martinez FA, et al. Randomised trial of losartan versus captopril in patients over 65 with heart failure (Evaluation of Losartan in the Elderly Study, ELITE). Lancet. 1997; 349:747–52.

42. Ruggenenti P, Fassi A, Ilieva A, et al. Effects of verapamil added-on trandolapril therapy in hypertensive type 2 diabetes patients with microalbuminuria: the BENEDICT-B randomized trial. J Hypertens. 2011;29:207–16.

43. Ruilope LM, Jakobsen A, Heroys J, et al. Prospects for renovascular protection by more aggressive renin-angiotensin system control. Medscape J Med. 2008;10(Suppl):S5.

44. Rutherford JD, Pfeffer MA, Moyè LA, et al. Effect of captopril on ischemic events after myocardial infarction. Results of the survival and ventricular enlargement trial. SAVE Investigators. Cirulation. 1994;90:1731–8.

45. Sanders GD, Coeytaux R, Dolor RJ, et al. Angiotensin-Converting Enzyme Inhibitors (ACEIs), Angiotensin II Receptor Antagonists (ARBs), and Direct Renin Inhibitors for Treating Essential Hypertension: An Update. Rockville (MD): Agency for Healthcare Research and Quality (US); 2011.
46. Savarese G, Costanzo P, Cleland JG, et al. A meta-analysis reporting effects of angiotensin-converting enzyme inhibitors and angiotensin receptor blockers in patients without heart failure. J Am Coll Cardiol. 2013;61:131–42.
47. Schmieder RE, Delles C, Mimran A, et al. Impact of telmisartan versus ramipril on renal endothelial function in patients with hypertension and type 2 diabetes. Diabetes Care. 2007;30:1351–6.
48. Schmieder RE, Hilgers KF, Schlaich MP, et al. Renin-angiotensin system and cardiovascular risk. Lancet. 2007;369:1208–19.
49. Schrader J, Luders S, Kulschewski A, et al. Morbidity and mortality after stroke, eprosartan compared with nitrendipine for secondary prevention: principal results of a prospective randomized controlled study (MOSES). Stroke. 2005;36:1218–26.
50. Strauss MH, Hall AS. Angiotensin receptor blockers may increase risk of myocardial infarction: unraveling the ARB-MI paradox. Circulation. 2006;114:838–54.
51. Swedberg K, Held P, Kjekshus J, et al. Effects of the early administration of enalapril on mortality in patients with acute myocardial infarction. Results of the Cooperative New Scandinavian Enalapril Survival Study II (CONSENSUS II). N Engl J Med. 1992;327:678–84.
52. The AIRE Study Investigators. Effect of ramipril on mortality and morbidity of survivors of acute myocardial infarction with clinical evidence of heart failure. Lancet. 1993;342:821–8.
53. The CONSENSUS Trial Study Group. Effects of enalapril on mortality in severe congestive heart failure. Results of the Cooperative North Scandinavian Enalapril Survival Study (CONSENSUS). N Engl J Med. 1987;316:1429–35.
54. The Editors of the Lancet. Retraction – Combination treatment of angiotensin-II receptor blocker and angiotensin-converting-enzyme inhibitor in non-diabetic renal disease (COOPERATE): a randomised controlled trial. Lancet. 2009;374:1226.
55. The SOLVD Investigators. Effect of enalapril on survival in patients with reduced left ventricular ejection fractions and congestive heart failure. N Engl J Med. 1991;325:293–302.
56. Turnbull F, Neal B, Pfeffer M, et al. Blood pressure-dependent and independent effects of agents that inhibit the renin-angiotensin system. J Hypertens. 2007;25:951–8.

57. van Vark LC, Bertrand M, Akkerhuis KM, et al. Angiotensin-converting enzyme inhibitors reduce mortality in hypertension: a meta-analysis of randomized clinical trials of renin-angiotensin-aldosterone system inhibitors involving 158,998 patients. Eur Heart J. 2012;33:2088–97.

58. Verdecchia P, Gentile G, Angeli F, et al. Beyond blood pressure: evidence for cardiovascular, cerebrovascular, and renal protective effects of renin-angiotensin system blockers. Ther Adv Cardiovasc Dis. 2012;6:81–91.

59. Viberti G, Wheeldon NM, MicroAlbuminuria Reduction With VSI. Microalbuminuria reduction with valsartan in patients with type 2 diabetes mellitus: a blood pressure-independent effect. Circulation. 2002;106:672–8.

60. Weir MR. Effects of renin-angiotensin system inhibition on end-organ protection: can we do better? Clin Ther. 2007;29:1803–24.

61. Wong J. Is there benefit in dual renin-angiotensin-aldosterone system blockade? No, yes and maybe: a guide for the perplexed. Diab Vasc Dis Res. 2013;10:193–201.

62. Yusuf S, Pfeffer MA, Swedberg K, et al. Effects of candesartan in patients with chronic heart failure and preserved left-ventricular ejection fraction: the CHARM-Preserved Trial. Lancet. 2003;362:777–81.

63. Yusuf S, Sleight P, Pogue J, et al. Effects of an angiotensin-converting-enzyme inhibitor, ramipril, on cardiovascular events in high-risk patients. The Heart Outcomes Prevention Evaluation Study Investigators. N Engl J Med. 2000;342:145–53.

64. Yusuf S, Teo K, Anderson C, et al. Effects of the angiotensin-receptor blocker telmisartan on cardiovascular events in high-risk patients intolerant to angiotensin-converting enzyme inhibitors: a randomised controlled trial. Lancet. 2008; 372:1174–83.

Index

A

ACE. *See* Angiotensin
converting enzyme (ACE)
ACE inhibitors (ACEIs), 1–30,
41–67, 74–83, 85, 91–94,
96–101, 103–104, 106, 120,
121, 123–128, 133–142
ACEIs. *See* ACE inhibitors
(ACEIs)
Acyltransferase-1 (AT1), 6, 7, 12,
25, 26, 53
Ang II. *See* Angiotensin II
(Ang II)
Angiotensin converting enzyme
(ACE), 2, 4, 9, 18, 21,
51–53, 120, 121, 127
Angiotensin II (Ang II), 1–3,
6–13, 15, 16, 18–24, 26, 28,
29, 51, 53–55, 121–122
Angiotensin II receptor blockers
(ARBs), 2–9, 11, 12, 17–22,
24–27, 29, 30, 52, 55, 61–62,
64, 74–76, 79–81, 85, 89,
91–94, 96, 97, 99, 101–104,
106, 120, 121, 128–142
Antihypertensive treatment,
5, 15, 74–76, 78, 81, 91,
94–106, 133

ARBs. *See* Angiotensin II
receptor blockers (ARBs)
AT1. *See* Acyltransferase-1
(AT1)
AT1 antagonists, 1–30

C

Cardiovascular (CV), 1–4, 7–9,
12, 15, 16, 19, 22, 24–29, 43,
58, 61, 62, 67, 73, 74, 79–83,
85–89, 91, 92, 95, 100,
104–106, 121–123, 127, 128,
133, 134, 139, 141, 142
Chronic kidney disease (CKD),
19–22, 73–106, 123, 133
CKD. *See* Chronic kidney disease
(CKD)
Clinical trials, 4, 6, 9, 17, 20, 29,
67, 75, 76, 104, 106, 120,
123–138
CV. *See* Cardiovascular (CV)

D

Diabetes, 1, 3, 5, 9–15, 20, 23, 54,
55, 58, 64, 65, 73–106, 123,
128, 139, 141, 142

© Springer International Publishing Switzerland 2015   149
P. Perrone Filardi (ed.), *ACEi and ARBS in Hypertension
and Heart Failure*, Current Cardiovascular Therapy 5,
DOI 10.1007/978-3-319-09788-6